UNDERSTAND[...]
AND THE MENOPAUSE

About the author

AFTER graduating from Aberdeen University, Scotland in 1956 with a Bachelor of Medicine and Surgery degree Robert Wilson set up in practice in Calgary, Alberta, Canada. He was awarded a Canadian MD degree as well as the Certificate of the College of Family Physicians of Canada.

In 1970 he was elected Vice-President of the Medical Staff at St Joseph's Hospital, London, Ontario and in 1974 he occupied a teaching position in medicine at the University of Western Ontario in the same city.

Dr Wilson's research into hormone and mood swings in relation to the menstrual cycle and the menopause began in 1978. He established a Clinic for Preventive Medicine in Vancouver, B.C. with University of British Columbia affiliation and held staff appointments at the University Hospital and at the Vancouver General Hospital. He has written two books on premenstrual syndrome, one published in Canada (*Controlling PMS*) and the other in the UK (*PMS – Diet Against It*). He is also the author of numerous articles published in medical journals in both Canada and the UK.

Dr Wilson currently consults on general preventive medicine at BUPA, and on the menopause and PMS in particular both at BUPA and at the Portland Hospital for Women and Children (both in London).

UNDERSTANDING HRT AND THE MENOPAUSE

DR ROBERT C D WILSON

CONSUMERS' ASSOCIATION

Which? Books are commissioned by
Consumers' Association and published by
Which? Ltd, 2 Marylebone Road, London NW1 4DF

Distributed by The Penguin Group:
Penguin Books Limited,
27 Wrights Lane, London W8 5TZ

First edition June 1992
Reprinted August 1992
Second edition 1995
Copyright © 1992, 1995 Which? Ltd

British Library Cataloguing in Publication Data
Wilson, Robert C. D.
   Understanding HRT and the Menopause
   I. Title
   618.1

ISBN 0-85202-572-6

Acknowledgements
Australian Consumers' Association for permission to use the table on skin
moisturisers on page 94. The table was first published in *Choice* magazine in
February 1982.
   CIBA for permission to use advice from the leaflet 'Helpful Hints on Using
Your Patch' and to recreate their illustrations.
   HMSO for permission to use the table on calcium content of foods on pages
107-8 which was abstracted from Paul, A. A. & Southgate, D. 1978. In
McCance and Widdowson's *The Composition of Foods*, 4th rev. ed. London.
   Women's Nationwide Cancer Control Campaign for permission to adapt
their material for the illustrations on pages 176-7.
   Proceedings of 8th Reinier de Graaf Symposium: 'Ovarian Endocrinopathies',
Amsterdam, September 1993 Excerpta Medica, for permission to include its
information on follicle xenografting (contained in Chapter 12).
   The *Financial Times* for permission to use information on gene medicine
supplied in 14 March 1995 edition (contained in Chapter 12).

Cover photograph by ACE, Mauritius
Cover design by Ridgeway Associates
Text illustrations by Stuart McLean
Typographic design by Paul Saunders
Typeset by FMT Graphics, London
Printed in England by Clays Ltd, Bungay, Suffolk

Contents

FOREWORD

MIDDLE age, menopause and HRT are much discussed by women among themselves and, if they have a sympathetic ear, with their GPs; but the side effects of the menopause, not experienced by everyone of course, are still all too often irritating, upsetting and even embarrassing. Or at least they have that reputation. *Woman's Hour* on BBC Radio 4, a programme with which I was associated for fifteen years, was one of the pioneers of sensible discussions of what menopause means – despite, in the programme's early years, unintentionally hilarious memos from BBC bosses about the unsuitability of any discussion of wombs and hot flushes at two o'clock in the afternoon. Fortunately in our more enlightened times menopause is no longer taboo, though sensible, reliable and up-to-date information about it and how to minimise its less appealing aspects hasn't been all that easy to find. This book offers a great deal of helpful information and guidance. Those who are members of the HRT 'club' can feel secure in their decision to join; those who've been advised not to (or prefer not to) use HRT can reconsider their decision from the evidence, or perhaps decide that they have after all made the correct decision. Above all this book should enable women to make an informed choice, and to know that the middle years can be positively enjoyed.

Sue MacGregor

AUTHOR'S NOTE

No book can be written without ideas. The inspiration for this work came from three eminent gynaecologists: Malcolm Whitehead of King's College Hospital; Adam Magos, of The Royal Free Hospital, and Miss Mary Anderson, of Harley Street, all of London.

I would like to thank the staff at the libraries of the College of Physicians and Surgeons of British Columbia, Vancouver, Canada and at the Royal Society of Medicine in London who have been so helpful during my research.

Many patients have lent their support to this book, in both enthusiasm and comment. To all of them my sincere thanks.

Finally, to my wife Maureen, who typed and retyped the manuscript, my deep gratitude and appreciation. Without her encouragement and devotion this book would not have been possible.

INTRODUCTION

THIS BOOK was written in response to the many women who complained to me in the late 'eighties and early 'nineties of the dearth of solid, forthright information concerning the menopause and surrounding years. Three eventful years have passed since the first edition. They say that in politics a week is a long time: in medicine much can happen in a single day. Advances in science proceed at such a pace that new discoveries are being made, somewhere, by someone, as each minute passes.

Research into the menopause is no exception. Magazines, newspapers and television programmes report daily upon the latest findings, often sensationally and without putting them into the context of the broad span of medical research. Yet the greater the knowledge of health indicators and predictors the better informed will be the decisions made by women and their physicians, especially concerning the modification and prevention of menopausal symptoms, cardiovascular disease, osteoporosis and cancer.

Hormone replacement therapy (HRT) affects health in ways that are interpreted differently by different experts. Some risks are reduced, others raised, and on others there is no consensus as yet. In this book, I have tried to explain HRT and the menopause in some detail, yet in simple enough terms for the information to be accessible to all women, whether or not they have any prior medical knowledge. This book also addresses the latest developments in gynaecology, which have been described in established medical journals or presented at international medical gatherings.

The word 'menopause' simply means cessation of the menses, or monthly periods. It is not a sudden event – indeed, the associated effects may last over 10 years – but it signals the end of a woman's reproductive years. The menopause takes place in three stages: the peri-menopause, the menopause and the post-menopause, which follow a sequential pattern and merge into each other. The three phases used to be collectively called the climacteric, a term now little used, but may be better known as the 'change of life' or simply 'the change'.

The peri-menopause signals declining function of the ovaries; during this stage menstruation usually becomes irregular and other symptoms such as hot flushes, night sweats and sleep disturbance are common. When there have been no menstrual periods for 12 months the post-menopausal stage has started and the menopause has taken place, a point signalled by the last menstrual period.

Psychological symptoms such as mood swings, anxiety, irritability, feelings of inadequacy, loss of energy and depression are common. There is, however, some doubt as to whether these are due to the ovaries ceasing to produce oestrogen or are the result of other problems such as sleep disturbance, hot flushes and social factors which may exacerbate pre-existing psychological problems.

It is true to say that in Western society the menopause is not generally regarded as a boon. While a few women are glad to be relieved of menstruation and the need for contraception, it is not surprising, given the importance that our society places upon youth and physical attractiveness, that many approach the menopause with a sense that life's doors are closing. There is a big difference between not wanting to become pregnant and being no longer physically able to do so; it may seem to some women that the ending of fertility represents the passing of a major element of their womanhood.

The attitude of society towards ageing women no doubt contributes to the feelings of unwantedness and depression that some women feel at this time. Attractive young women are seen as a desirable asset. They are used by the media to sell clothes, cars, maga- zines and all manner of other consumer goods. The status of many an overweight, balding middle-aged man has been greatly enhanced in the eyes of his peers by the acquisition of a young and glamorous girlfriend. But what of the older woman? The term 'menopausal woman' is used as an expression of dismissive contempt. Research has shown that middle-aged and older women find it harder to get service in shops and restaurants; they are simply not noticed. If they have had a family, their children are probably at an age where they want complete independence from their parents. It is small wonder that many women experience a feeling of worthlessness; they are losing their role as a physically desirable and fertile woman and the new status facing them seems unattractive in the extreme. Added to this, they have the physiological symptoms of the menopause to contend with. The phrase 'change of life' seems all too apt.

Yet there have never been more examples among us of women in their forties and fifties – and beyond – who are attractive, confident and assertive, who get a lot out of life and make a valuable contribution to it. They are the very antithesis of the image that society has thrust upon them.

The number of women who are post-menopausal is rapidly increasing. Improvements in diet, medical care, general health and lifestyle are resulting in a far greater number of women living to a far greater age than a century ago. By the turn of the century about 14 million women in the United Kingdom will be post-menopausal.

During the last 100 years the average life expectancy of women in Britain has risen progressively from 50 years in 1900 to 62 years in 1940 and now, in the 1990s, to nearly 83 years. Over the same period, the number of fertile years has changed little. The onset of menstruation now takes place at approximately 13 years, as opposed to the average of 17 years 50 to 60 years ago; interestingly, however, the time of the last menstrual period does not appear to have altered over the centuries, usually occurring between the ages of 49 and 51. Hence, a woman who lives to 80 or beyond will have spent more than one-third of her life in the post-menopausal state.

Hormone replacement therapy is now an option for all women who are approaching the menopause, and for its many advocates it is life-transforming. It is not a 'fountain of youth' but it does help to maintain skin elasticity and bone density, it facilitates an active sex life and it creates an improved sense of well-being. It also keeps down the level of fats in the blood and may reduce the risk of clotting. Over the last twenty years it has become apparent that women undergoing HRT have suffered fewer heart attacks, strokes and less osteoporosis ('brittle bones', liable to fracture easily) than those who were not. But it may not suit all women: some menopausal women may be advised by their GP not to take it because of existing medical conditions. What is more, there are many different forms of HRT, and it is important that the treatment is individually tailored to those women who opt for it.

Among the many questions that may come to mind when women are considering the pros and cons of hormone replacement therapy are:

- Is it true that night sweats and hot flushes can be avoided if I take HRT?
- How likely am I to suffer from osteoporosis/heart disease/breast cancer/endometrial cancer if I choose – or choose not – to take HRT?
- Do I need dietary supplements during the menopause?
- What is the most appropriate method of contraception in my situation?
- What effect will HRT have on my sex drive?
- Should I expect to suffer from other disorders and problems, such as depression, varicose veins and recurrent thrush and cystitis?
- For how long should I expect to undergo HRT? Am I starting on a regime for the rest of my life?
- Can HRT be addictive?
- Given that HRT is relatively new and given that there are so many different preparations on the market, how can I be sure that I am getting the best treatment?
- I was on the Pill for many years and I feel I don't want to keep taking hormones all my life. What alternative methods are there to get me through the menopause comfortably?
- Thirty years ago the Pill was considered to be the answer to all our problems, but there were lots of scares about it later. If I go on HRT will I be a guinea-pig for future generations?
- How can I be sure that if I go on HRT I won't develop some medical problem when I'm 80 that no one yet knows about?
- How will I actually *feel* during the menopause?

This book will answer such queries.

Notable changes for this edition are:
- a new chapter (4) on cardiovascular disease, the leading cause of death in women: despite the fact that it is more prevalent in women than any form of cancer, there is evidence to suggest that women are referred later than men for investigative procedures. Research indicates that oestrogen replacement therapy reduces by about 40 per cent the risk of cardiovascular disease

- expansion of the chapter (3) on osteoporosis to include beneficial non-hormone therapies for prevention and treatment of the condition. After the age of 35 bone density decreases until the menopause, at which point falling oestrogen levels accelerate the condition. A 50-year-old woman has a 15 per cent lifetime probability of an osteoporotic hip fracture
- a new chapter (6) on the risks associated with HRT, focussing in particular on breast cancer. At age 50 a woman has a 10 per cent probability of developing breast cancer and a 3 per cent probability of dying from the disease. The median age of development is 69 years, but women are living longer: as we approach the millennium life expectancy is 80 years plus. One-third of a women's expected lifespan is post-menopausal, allowing more time, therefore, for breast cancer to become evident. Women at high risk of developing breast cancer are identifiable, as are family members at risk of carrying a breast cancer gene. The preventive capabilities of the drug tamoxifen, anti-oxidants and retinoids are reviewed in this chapter. However, the control of breast cancer through prevention remains dependent on knowledge of the cause
- major expansion of the chapter (5) on HRT: new preparations are discussed, including dosage and side effects, and current trials for the convenient HRT nasal spray ('the sniff') described. As ever, finding the right combination of oestrogen and progestogen is the key to safe and successful use of HRT. Time and perseverance are necessary on the part of both patient and doctor if the right balance of hormones – one which will not have adverse effects on blood lipids, blood coagulability or mood – is achieved
- expansion where appropriate in all the remaining chapters in the light of international research: contraception, screening and in particular new developments in mammography are closely scrutinised. Advances in the prevention of connective tissue urinary disorders, the link between oestrogen lack and loss of memory, and the reason why certain stress-related disorders become more evident at the menopause, are also explained
- the final chapter (12) looks to a future in which gene hunters and gene medicine will be the key forces in the fight against illness.

With the extension of the normal lifespan, healthy ageing opens new doors for women. Decisions taken now can make a remarkable difference to the quality of the years ahead – years that can be rewarding, enjoyable and fulfilling in different ways.

This book enables women to make the right decisions. It helps them to recognise menopausal symptoms; understand the benefits (and possible drawbacks) of hormone replacement therapy; establish a healthy lifestyle by means of good nutrition, adequate exercise and stress management; and choose the right contraception for the menopausal years. In other words, it will put them in a much stronger position to take responsibility for the key decisions of their personal health management. By reading and learning all they can about this phase of their lives they will be able to maximise their enjoyment of the future.

Robert C. D. Wilson

CHAPTER 1

THE MENSTRUAL CYCLE

AT PUBERTY, a major internal bio-chemical change is evidenced by an external physical event. Some of the chemicals responsible are hormones, which are released from the pituitary gland situated in the brain. Part of it, the hypothalamus, regulates the amount of hormones released from the pituitary gland. The two key hormones are follicle-stimulating hormone (FSH) and luteinising hormone (LH), collectively known as gonadotrophins. These are the nourishing hormones that stimulate the ovaries to produce two further hormones, oestrogen and progesterone.

Puberty begins when oestrogen floods into the bloodstream, causing early budding of breast tissue, influencing the development of fat deposits and smoothing the body contours to produce the characteristic female outline. Pubic and underarm hair begins to grow, and special sweat glands, the apocrine glands, located at the entrance to the vagina and anus, under the arms and around the nipples and navel, start to function. While ordinary sweat glands exude an odourless combination of sweat, water and lactic acid, the apocrine glands exude a milky liquid with a characteristic odour. Oestrogen also causes enlargement of the ovaries, from the size of a grape to that of a walnut, which takes 12-24 months following the onset of puberty. The ovaries are then ready for egg production.

Under the influence of follicle-stimulating hormone and luteinising hormone from the pituitary gland the first menstruation, or 'menarche', occurs. This represents a major change: a step from girlhood to womanhood. The time of the menarche varies and seems to be influenced by factors such as race, genes, diet and socio-economic background.

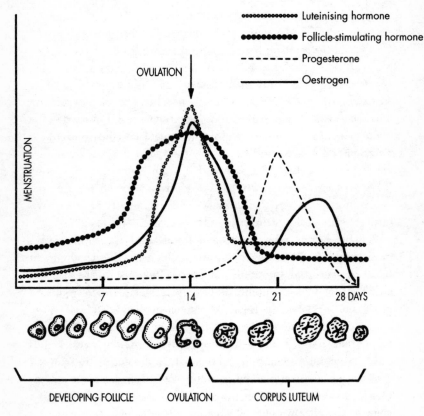

Figure 1   Hormone changes during the menstrual cycle

During the first year following the menarche it is normal for only three or four episodes of menstruation (periods) to occur, lasting on average five to six days. During the early teens periods become more frequent. Menstruation usually takes place every one or two months and lasts for five days. Thereafter a regular cycle will establish itself.

The normal cycle

The reproductive cycle normally lasts an average of 28 days, though it can range from 20 to 36 days. The duration of the menstrual flow may also change from month to month, lasting from two to eight days. Such a range is perfectly normal. The amount of blood lost can also vary a good deal, from 50 to 175 cc; average loss is under 120 cc per month.

The first 14 days of the cycle are known as the proliferative phase and the last 14 days, from ovulation to the onset of menstruation, the secretory phase (see figure 1).

Ovulation

Within about two years of puberty the process of ovulation begins. At birth the ovaries contain approximately two million immature egg cells, called oocytes. By the menarche only some 300,000 remain, the others having been lost over the years through natural attrition (atresia). A minimum of 1,000 egg cells is thought to be required for the maintenance of the menstrual cycle. At the menarche the follicle-stimulating hormone causes egg cells to mature, usually one at a time. Each egg cell is situated in a follicle in the ovary. These ovarian follicles are lined with granulosa cells, and it is these cells that produce the hormone oestrogen, which, when released into the bloodstream, has a powerful effect on the lining of the uterus (the endometrium). The lining thickens and becomes rich in blood vessels: this is the proliferative phase. The ripening egg cell has meanwhile pushed its way to the surface of the ovary, where it produces a blister which ruptures, and releases the egg into the Fallopian tube. Ovulation has then taken place.

This event is caused by a surge in the amount of the luteinising hormone from the pituitary gland. Recent research has shown that the granulosa cells of the ovarian follicle produce, in addition to

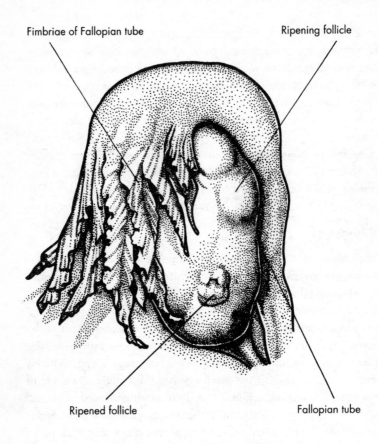

Fimbriae of Fallopian tube

Ripening follicle

Ripened follicle

Fallopian tube

Figure 2   The ovary and follicle

oestrogen, a protein-like substance called inhibin. The rising level of inhibin in the bloodstream reduces the amount of the follicle-stimulating hormone secretion from the pituitary, and this in turn initiates the luteinising hormone surge which induces ovulation.

At the burst follicle, granulosa cells accumulate and fold inwards upon themselves, to form a yellow-pink structure (corpus luteum) on the surface of the ovary. This is the source of the second ovarian hormone, progesterone. Progesterone causes the new tissue of the endometrium, which was laid down under the direction of oestrogen during the proliferative phase, to become softer and sponge-like (secretory phase), ready to receive a fertilised egg.

The walls of the vagina are kept moist by mucus-producing cells. During the proliferative phase, the oestrogen produced by the ovary causes the mucus to be thin, watery and clear, assisting the passage of any sperm towards the Fallopian tubes leading from the uterus. In the secretory phase, after ovulation, the progesterone produced from the corpus luteum causes the vaginal mucus to thicken and become more tenacious. This altered mucus hinders further sperm from entering the Fallopian tubes. Both oestrogen and progesterone tend to cause wave-like contractions in the tubes, assisting the egg in its average six-and-a-half-day voyage to the uterus.

If a sperm and egg unite conception takes place and the fertilised egg (ovum) then travels to the uterus, where it embeds itself in the soft endometrial layer. The delicate communication system that links the hypothalamus, pituitary, ovary and uterus is now activated, with the result that the level of progesterone is increased, and maintained, to ensure the health of the endometrium. Continued progesterone production by the ovary is assured with the formation of a corpus luteum cyst at, or near, the site of the ruptured ovarian follicle. After about the ninth week of pregnancy, the progesterone produced from this cyst is topped up by additional progesterone production from the developing placenta. This nourishing/receiving pad at the end of the umbilical cord delivers nourishment to the foetus.

Research indicates that an adequate blood level of the hormone prolactin is necessary for normal corpus luteal function, further progesterone production, and the maintenance of a healthy pregnancy. Exactly how prolactin influences the normal menstrual cycle is as yet unclear, but it is known that the hypothalamus regulates its production, and release, by the pituitary gland.

Menstruation

If conception does not take place the ovary continues to produce progesterone and oestrogen until approximately the 24th day of the cycle. At this point the communication mechanism is again activated by the falling oestrogen and progesterone levels. The hypothalamus reduces its controlling releasing hormone to the pituitary gland, which in turn decreases the supply of follicle-stimulating hormone and luteinising hormone to the ovary. Consequently, during the last three days of the cycle there is a dramatic reduction in both oestrogen and progesterone which causes a decrease in blood flow to the uterus. Cell destruction results, and the unnourished uterine lining is shed. The menstrual flow begins as the unwanted endometrium is discarded.

Menstruation is often accompanied by cramps – contractions of the muscle wall of the uterus as it squeezes the endometrium free and assists in its expulsion. The damaged endometrial cells release hormone-like substances called prostaglandins. These have been shown to be of immense importance in the overall balance mechanism of the body (see Chapter 7).

The peri-menopausal cycle

During the fertile years there is a gradual depletion of ovarian follicles, and hence the egg cells they contain. The loss of egg cells (follicles) accelerates once the number has fallen below 25,000 (usually around the age of 35). If this were not so, the menopause would not happen until about age 70.

It is thought that if 90 per cent of ovary tissue were not functioning at the age of 16 the menopause would occur at 28 years. If one ovary has to be removed at age 30, the menopause would probably start at 44.

The reason for the acceleration of egg cell disappearance may be genetic (Turner's syndrome) or age-related; it can also be caused by radiation treatment, chemotherapy, disease or toxins (mumps oöphoritis and cigarette-smoking), or by surgery.

At the menopause only a few eggs remain. With the depletion of the follicles, the level of fertility is reduced and oestrogen deficiency begins. As the number of granulosa cells in the follicles reduces, inhibin production also decreases, very gradually. The level of follicle-stimulating hormone therefore changes little.

By the early forties the number of granulosa cells has decreased to such a degree that the level of inhibin they secrete will have fallen to a critical point; the level of follicle-stimulating hormone now rises. Although the menstrual periods may still be completely regular and no menopausal symptoms are being experienced, the rising follicle-stimulating hormone level represents the beginning of the peri-menopause.

As follicle depletion continues over the next few years the level of follicle-stimulating hormone will fluctuate, causing the menstrual cycle to become irregular. The amount of menstrual flow also alters, being sometimes lighter and sometimes heavier. By now the follicle-stimulating hormone will be approaching, or have reached, the point at which the peri-menopause can be said to have begun. Conception is now unlikely to happen. Oestrogen production usually remains near-normal in the early years of the peri-menopause, therefore symptoms associated with oestrogen deficiency, such as hot flushes and vaginal dryness, will not yet be evident. As oestrogen levels fall over the next few years the occasional hot flush, increasing tiredness and perhaps dizziness will occur, and menstrual periods may become more irregular with episodes of heavy bleeding.

The menopause

The menopause has been reached when there has been no bleeding for 12 months. This indicates that there is no longer any stimulation of the endometrium by the two ovarian hormones oestrogen and progesterone, but it does not mean that the body is producing no oestrogen at all; it is still produced (in small quantities) by the post-menopausal ovaries and from the adrenal glands, which are situated on top of each kidney. Another source of oestrogen is androstenedione. This weak androgen steroid is converted in the liver, and in fat tissue, to a weak form of oestrogen called oestrone. However, oestrone production rarely reaches sufficient quantity to prevent menopausal symptoms and signs (further information follows in Chapter 2).

The menopause tends to take place between the ages of 45 and 54, and especially between 49 and 51. It is likely to happen about two years earlier in cigarette-smokers and in women who have had a hysterectomy without removal of both ovaries.

A few women may cease to menstruate in their thirties. The egg cells within the ovaries disappear spontaneously, causing sudden cessation of menstruation and abrupt hormonal changes. The reason for premature menopause is not always known, but contributory factors are listed on page 20. The loss of ovarian hormones creates a risk of osteoporosis as well as hot flushes, vaginal changes and psychological symptoms, just as in a normal menopause.

Sometimes an artificial menopause is induced when a woman's ovaries are removed surgically or irradiated. The egg cells are destroyed and again the menopause begins suddenly with the same attendant effects. Hysterectomy (removal of the uterus) without removal of the ovaries before the menopause is now considered to accelerate the onset of ovarian failure by about two years.

The ovarian hormones

The two significant female ovarian hormones, oestrogen and progesterone, have a profound effect on the body. During the perimenopause, and at the menopause, the changes that take place are due in particular to a lack of these two hormones.

Oestrogen
Oestrogen attaches itself to the surface of cells and in organs where it is needed, influencing the functioning of that organ either by its presence (during the fertile years) or by its absence (after the menopause). The chief source of oestrogen is the granulosa cells.

Table 1: What does oestrogen do?
1 Maintains the health and proper functioning of the genital organs
2 Causes the endometrium (uterus lining) to thicken in the proliferative phase of the menstrual cycle
3 Softens the cervix and produces the thin mucus in which the sperm can swim
4 Enhances the chance of fertilisation by improving the mobility of the egg as it passes down the Fallopian tubes
5 Acts with inhibin to affect the hypothalamus in its regulation of the menstrual cycle
6 Acts with prostaglandins (hormone-like substances) to maintain the

health of the walls of blood vessels

7 Maintains supply of collagen to the skin, which promotes skin elasticity, and calcium to the bones, which keeps them strong

8 Influences the development of the breasts and maintains breast structure and the milk ducts

9 Affects the thickness of the skin and the condition of the hair

10 Causes the emergence of typical female shape and form at puberty

11 Brings about the energy, happy disposition and positive outlook often typical of the first two weeks, in particular, of the menstrual cycle

Progesterone

The second female hormone produced by the ovary is progesterone, which is broken down by the liver and secreted in the urine as pregnanediol. This corpus luteum hormone, of equal importance to oestrogen, has recently been linked with it in a preventive role against osteoporosis. Synthetic progesterone (progestogen) is used with natural oestrogens for the control of menopausal symptoms.

Table 2: What does progesterone do?

1 Transforms the proliferative endometrium to the secretory form in the second half of the menstrual cycle

2 Changes the cervical mucus in the second half of the menstrual cycle from a thin and watery substance to one which is thicker and tenacious

3 Tends to reduce the acidity level of the vagina

4 Joins with oestrogen to lower the levels of follicle-stimulating hormone and luteinising hormone by acting with inhibin on the hypothalamus

5 Raises the basal body temperature, which can be measured at the time of ovulation

6 Maintains pregnancy through an intricate hormonal interaction

7 Stimulates development of breast tissue, particularly the alveoli gland system

8 Encourages water and salt retention (although less so than synthetic progestogen)

9 Enhances the immune system through intricate links with prostaglandins and immunoglobulins

10 Influences mood during the latter half of the menstrual cycle

Premenstrual syndrome

Research indicates that the physical and mood changes that occur before menstruation result from the imbalance between oestrogen and progesterone which occurs at this time. They are known as premenstrual syndrome (PMS), a complex disorder for which commonly reported symptoms include fatigue, headache, backache, aggression, depression, irritability, mood swings, weight gain, skin eruptions, food craving, feelings of bloatedness, and sore breasts. It is not unusual for PMS to worsen slightly in the peri-menopause, probably owing to the increasing fluctuations in the relationship between oestrogen and progesterone at this time of life.

Relaxation techniques for stress management, exercise and changes to the diet often help women with mild symptoms to cope. Studies of the association of levels of blood progesterone and blood sugar have suggested that low blood sugar levels, which may occur during long intervals between meals, can result in the release of adrenalin. Progesterone is prevented by adrenalin from being taken up by its receptor, which can further upset the chemical balance between oestrogen and progesterone and cause other chemicals (neutrotransmitters) to be released in the brain, altering mood and behaviour.

As ovulation becomes less frequent, progesterone is not produced from the ovary in sufficient quantity to override the endometrium build-up. Consequently, when it is produced, the shedding of the excessive thickened endometrium will be heavier than usual, and its timing unpredictable (dysfunctional bleeding). The lowered progesterone level may further aggravate pre-existing PMS, or initiate it on the run-up to the menopause.

Testosterone

This primary male hormone is produced in small quantities in women by both the ovaries and the adrenal glands. If too much is produced it may cause masculinisation and give rise to an excess of unwanted hair (hirsutism).

In post-menopausal women the ovary tends to produce more testosterone than in pre-menopausal years and this may explain why older women tend to show a degree of defeminisation and hirsutism.

The post-menopausal ovary is hormonally active for several years after the menopause. One function is to produce a small indirect amount of oestrogen (estradiol) from testosterone by a chemical process called aromatisation. The oestrogen thus produced may help to protect the vagina and parts of the urethra from early atrophy.

CHAPTER 2

SYMPTOMS AND SIGNS OF THE MENOPAUSE

THE TERMS 'symptoms' and 'signs' are often used interchangeably, but strictly speaking a symptom is a complaint of which the patient is herself aware whereas a sign, in medical terms, is determined by medical examination: for example, raised blood pressure, or altered cholesterol level.

As ovarian follicles become fewer in number so the amount of circulating 17B-oestradiol, the isolated form of oestrogen produced by the granulosa cells, falls, and symptoms of oestrogen deficiency become more evident. In overweight women, however, such symptoms are lessened (although not prevented) by the presence of oestrone, a weaker oestrogen which is produced by conversion of androstenedione in fatty tissues.

Oestrogen deficiency is linked with, but not always entirely responsible for, the various symptoms and signs which occur around the menopause. However, about 20 per cent of women may experience few or none of these symptoms, which may be considered as physical, psychological or sexual.

Physical symptoms

Altered menstrual flow

During the peri-menopause menstrual flow may alter in both volume and duration, which signals changes taking place in the control mechanism between the hypothalamus and the pituitary gland. While irregular periods are quite normal, irregular bleeding is not; any bleeding that occurs between periods, after intercourse or after the menopause needs medical investigation.

Dysfunctional uterine bleeding – erratic and irregular *menstrual* bleeding – is often heavy and also requires medical attention to bring it under control. Simple medication is usually sufficient, but possible causes other than the menopause have first to be ruled out, perhaps by exploratory procedures such as endometrial biopsy or dilatation and curettage (see Chapter 10), as well as by blood tests.

Painful periods

Pain associated with normal or abnormal menstrual bleeding is known as dysmenorrhoea. It may be caused by infection, fibroids, endometriosis or prostaglandin imbalance (see Chapter 9).

Genital changes

The vagina, uterus and cervix (see figure 3) are areas where oestrogen is readily taken up and which consequently suffer when deficiency occurs: their lining, or surface tissue, then tends to atrophy. The vagina shortens, the skin surface weakens and thins and blood supply diminishes. Vaginal acidity lessens and dryness occurs as a result of a reduction in mucus glands, giving rise to painful intercourse, the risk of bleeding, and infection. Shrinkage of the uterus and cervix, together with shortening of the cervical canal, also takes place.

The bladder and urethra (the tube leading from the bladder to the outside of the body) are also affected, for they originally developed in the embryo in tandem with the genital tract. The lining walls shrink and become thinner and drier, hence more likely to crack and split and more vulnerable to infection. The trigone bladder (doorkeeper to the urethra) also atrophies, causing a pressing need to pass urine, and to pass it frequently, and sometimes incontinence after sneezing or coughing. Urge incontinence – an involuntary loss of urine which may occur with the sudden urge to urinate – responds well to exercises which can improve the surrounding muscles (see Chapter 9), while stress incontinence – involuntary loss of a little urine on coughing, sneezing or laughing – may require surgical correction (see Chapter 10).

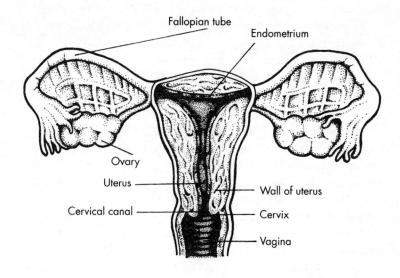

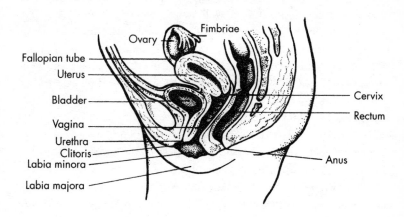

Figure 3   Female reproductive system

Skin and hair changes

'There is no magician's mantle to compare with the skin in its diverse roles of waterproof, overcoat, sunshade, suit of armour, and refrigeration, sensitive to the touch of a feather, and executing its own running repairs,' observes Professor R. D. Lockhart, anatomist, of Aberdeen University.

The skin constitutes the largest organ of the body. It is restless, constantly shedding its surface and repairing itself. It contains sweat glands, oil glands and hair follicles. Collagen and elastic fibres define its quality and support it.

At the peri-menopause an increasing dryness and thinning of the skin, brittle nails and changes to the hair may be noticed. Thirty per cent of skin collagen, which forms a large part of the connective support tissue of the skin, is lost in the first 10 years after the menopause; this causes further thinning of the skin, which increases the incidence of bruising and gives a transparent, waxy appearance.

Oestrogen replacement has been shown to restore lost collagen to pre-menopausal levels within six months, due in part to the fact that there are oestrogen receptors in the fibroblast cells (see Glossary) from which skin connective tissue is developed. It increases the water content of the skin as well as improving its blood flow. As women age, glandular function often becomes less efficient, which gives rise to dryness of the throat and burning of the eyes and mouth. Bowel upsets and constipation may also occur. All of these are caused by lack of water in the tissue combined with reduced blood supply. The body also absorbs calcium from food less well. Again, oestrogen can help.

Hair roots originate from the deep layers of skin connective tissue and are therefore affected by lack of oestrogen. Thicker, healthier hair is another benefit to be gained from oestrogen.

The actual growth of hair depends more on male hormones than oestrogen, which mainly affects the distribution of hair. As oestrogen levels fall the concentration of the sex hormone binding globulin is reduced and male hormones (androgens) increase, stimulating hair growth on the upper body and face.

Vasomotor symptoms (flushes, sweats and palpitations)

Vasomotor symptoms are those caused by the changing size of blood vessels, triggered by fluctuating oestrogen levels before the menopause. The commonest menopausal symptoms, experienced to some degree by 80 per cent of women, are vasomotor ones – hot flushes ('flashes' in North America), night sweats, palpitations and headaches (usually caused by lack of sleep resulting from the flushes and sweating, but not a primary menopausal symptom in themselves). New studies for which women's progress through the menopause has been tracked show that 40-58 per cent experience hot flushes within the two-year timespan surrounding their final menstrual period. Symptoms continue for more than a year in most women and for longer than five years in 29-50 per cent. Hot flushes usually start as a pressure sensation in the head followed by a feeling of heat which may extend from the head to the neck, upper chest and back, then spread to the whole body. In time, unlike other menopausal complaints, vasomotor symptoms decrease.

The exact cause of a hot flush is unknown, but there is a probable link with breakdown in the temperature control by the hypothalamus as oestrogen production declines during the peri-menopause. This in turn influences the sympathetic nervous system which dilates the blood vessels and gives rise to an increased heart rate (palpitations), and sometimes headaches. Brain chemicals called catecholamines and opiates are also thought to influence the heat regulatory mechanism, which is situated in the hypothalamus.

Oestrogen therapy helps to control the hormone level fluctuations, usually easing vasomotor symptoms within 10 days of treatment, although it may be two or three months before the full benefits are felt. Non-hormonal approaches which may help are reviewed in Chapter 7. Vasomotor symptoms are most noticeable just before and at the menopause, but then disappear as hormone levels stabilise.

Breast changes

The breasts develop at puberty under the influence of oestrogen. Around the menopause some gradual change may be apparent due to the reduction of both oestrogen and progesterone. The breasts may

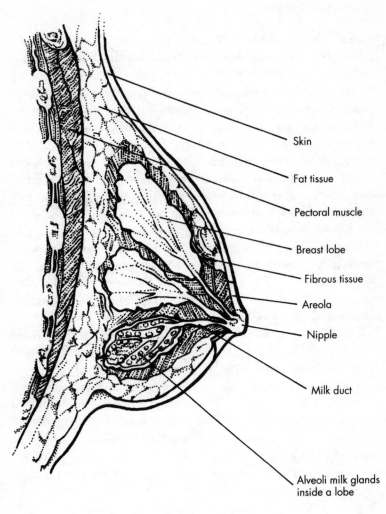

Skin

Fat tissue

Pectoral muscle

Breast lobe

Fibrous tissue

Areola

Nipple

Milk duct

Alveoli milk glands
inside a lobe

Figure 4   Structure of the breast

become smaller, with the nipples also reducing and becoming flatter and the areola darkening slightly; there may also be some roughness and thinning of the skin. (See figure 4.)

Bone and cardiovascular changes

Both bone and blood vessels undergo change at and after the menopause. Bone mass reduces more rapidly than during the peri-menopause and heart disease, in particular, is more likely to develop. These problems are considered at greater length in the chapters that follow.

Psychological symptoms

Emotional changes are commonly complained of by women experiencing the menopause. They include mood swings, irritability, anxiety, a poor memory, lack of concentration, feelings of inadequacy, loss of energy, tiredness and depression.

Whether the increase of psychological symptoms at this stage in life is due to a lack of oestrogen or the consequence of factors such as hot flushes, sleep disturbance and social influences is not known. It is possible that pre-existing psychological or psychiatric problems worsen at this time, aggravating mood change. According to the 'domino theory', loss of sleep caused by hot flushes and night-time wakefulness will give rise to fatigue, irritability and other alterations in normal functioning.

It was suggested in a 1986 study that beliefs held before the menopause about the experience of it may influence the individual's emotional symptoms during these years. Other research confirms that oestrogen exerts a direct 'mental tonic' effect that helps to counteract irritability, fatigue, insomnia, anxiety and depression.

Socio-economic factors

It has been shown that women of lower socio-economic groups have more psychological menopausal problems than those who are educated, financially secure, with pleasant homes, regular holidays and, possibly, rewarding jobs and/or sympathetic partners. The woman who is tired and overworked, with poor living conditions, financial worries and an inadequate diet, who has had little education and whose understanding of health matters is minimal, who has limited access to information, fears the unknown, feels inadequate and has a partner who finds it difficult to comprehend her menopause-related problems, may well have more difficulties in coming to terms with the 'change of life'.

Similarly, it may be perceived that a mature woman who has not had to face, as mothers do, the experience of offspring leaving home and the consequent 'empty nest' syndrome, with its attendant feelings of uselessness and unwantedness, may exhibit fewer psychological symptoms during the menopause. But there is no set pattern and the subject is a complex one.

Cultural attitudes

In Western society ageing generally and the menopause in particular are regarded negatively in the main. The anticipation of menopausal problems may therefore magnify their occurrence.

In other cultures age is revered and associated with wisdom. Consequently the menopause is welcomed as a positive event, bringing as it does an increase in status. This can be seen among certain castes in Rajasthan, for example, where the cessation of menstruation signals a woman's emergence from purdah, allowing her to mix freely with the male sex and to counsel younger members of her community. In Sub-Saharan Africa and Ethiopia post-menopausal women are accorded great respect and special status. Of course, in such Third World societies life expectancy is substantially lower, at about 40 to 50 years, than in industrialised countries, and contraception is not practised, so the women will have spent much of their time since puberty either pregnant or giving birth, which are potentially risky experiences in themselves. Therefore simply to reach the menopause confers status in a way which could not happen outside the Third World, and it may indeed be the last pregnancy which marks the point of transition to the menopause.

Western society, on the other hand, pursues the cult of youth and universally glorifies the desirability of the younger female at the expense of the mature woman. Faced with images of unattainable youthfulness throughout the media and society's preference for youth in most other areas of life, including the job market, the prospect of the menopause may seem to the middle-aged woman like a brutal reminder that the 'best' years of her life are now behind her.

But though her life may have changed in many ways it is likely to bring new opportunities and challenges. Some women change direction in their careers. Some start businesses or, free from the demands of raising their families, take an active role in their partner's career. Some re-direct their attention from the care of their children to the care of their elderly parents. For many, the approach of the menopause is a time for reflection and for reassessment of life's goals. Putting life into perspective will greatly assist the self-management of menopausal symptoms and is essential if a positive outlook is to be developed.

Personality and the link with depression

A woman's personality will influence the way in which she responds to the hormonal changes taking place at the menopause. Positive attitudes and high self-esteem will help to minimise the psychological effects of its physical symptoms.

It is an interesting fact that from puberty onwards women suffer from depression and anxiety disorders two to three times more often than do men, and that at times of marked hormonal change – premenstrually, post-natally and around the menopause – this tendency to depression is heightened. The psychological symptoms of the menopause may in fact represent a continuation and extension of premenstrual syndrome, albeit in an exaggerated form. However, this cannot be interpreted as being solely hormone-related, as psychological and other factors play a part.

In view of the variable and increasing hormone swings that take place approximately 10 years before the menopause, and for some years afterwards, it is quite probable that the balance between oestrogen and progesterone influences the intricate web of chemical messengers in the brain. These in turn initiate the physical and psychological symptoms, and in particular depression, which some women experience. Recent research in the United States indicates a potential link between a brain chemical, corticotrophin release hormone (CRH), oestrogen and susceptibility to depression. A gene has been located which produces this hormone when activated by oestrogen. The hormone appears to be pivotal in the way the body responds to stress, whether physical or mental, by co-ordinating these responses. It is thought that oestrogen controls, to some degree, the amount of CRH produced, and this influences the supply of other brain chemicals, such as serotonin. These substances have the ability to alter mood. This goes some way to explaining the link between oestrogen and mood disorders such as depression, anorexia nervosa and panic attacks (see also Chapter 7).

There is, however, more than one type of depression.

Depressed mood – low spirits, sadness or despondency are common symptoms around the menopause and are considered to be caused by lack of oestrogen. Depressed mood may be a response to hot flushes, sweats or disturbed sleep. Oestrogen therapy can be of assistance, but it is interesting to note that in some studies there are indications that oestrogen is no better than a placebo.

Depressive disorder can exist quite independently of the menopause, and is quite different from 'depressed mood'. Its symptoms are lack of concentration and interest, loss of appetite, weight and sex drive, feelings of impending doom, guilt and worthlessness, slow and quiet speech, early-morning waking and an inability to take decisions.

Depressive disorder, which is both far more serious and far more debilitating than depressed mood, is not common at the menopause, nor have studies revealed any relationship between the menopause and depressive disorder. Depressive disorder is usually treated with anti-depressant medication together with talking therapies.

Current research by Dr Barbara Sherwin at the University of McGill in Montreal links low levels of oestrogen to high levels of another brain neurotransmitter – monoamine oxidase. High levels of this substance cause a reduction in serotonin, deficiency in which can cause depression.

Dr Sherwin has also shown that oestrogen has a direct effect on memory function in certain aspects. There could be a link between lack of oestrogen and Alzheimer's disease, and if the hormone is linked with this form of brain dysfunction those menopausal women who have a family history of the disease would have good reason to consider hormone replacement therapy.

Sexual symptoms

Complex biological, emotional and social factors influence sexual behaviour. Sexual difficulties are common during the peri-menopausal years and may include poor sexual response, discomfort during intercourse, reduced libido and loss of interest in the sexual partner.

The mechanism of the sexual response is complicated and involves not only the body's reaction to touch and erotic stimulation but also the mental and emotional awareness of the partner's feelings. Gentleness, tenderness and consideration on the part of the partner will be of immense benefit at this time.

Oestrogen, when plentiful, maintains the size, shape, skin thickness and flexibility of the vagina and profoundly influences response to touch through its effect on skin sensation, lubrication and blood supply. Insufficient oestrogen can cause changes that make sexual intercourse uncomfortable, painful or even impossible. An understanding partner will appreciate that the vaginal dryness (resulting from lowered oestrogen levels) associated with the menopause will take longer to overcome during foreplay (the best method of lubrication yet devised). But if the difficulties are more severe it is well worth discussing them with a doctor so that they can be dealt with at an early stage.

Oestrogen rejuvenates the vagina, making it thicker, more flexible

Table 3: Orgasmic response

Age group	Sufficient natural lubrication %	Orgasm achieved in all age groups
50s	48	Most times with intercourse or with masturbation
60s	35	50 per cent of time with intercourse alone
70s	23	

Table 4: Sexual frequency

Age group	Sexually active %	Sexual activity at least once each week %
50+	88	73
60+	63	63
70+	50	50

Self-stimulation was reported by 47 per cent of all women respondents in their 50s, 37 per cent in their 60s and 37 per cent in their 70s

and more moist, but by no means all women need oestrogen replacement to maintain good sexual function after the menopause. An active sex life in itself plays a major role in keeping the sexual organs in good condition.

Table 3 shows the results of a Consumers Union study of orgasmic response among 1,844 American women in different age groups. Table 4 reveals the findings of a further study by Consumers Union among a similar number of women to investigate patterns of sexual activity. Of those interviewed, 75 per cent were married.

Beyond the age of 50 an increasing percentage of women cease all forms of sexual activity. This may be due to the fact that 50 per cent of women in this age group live alone and have difficulty finding partners. Ill-health may reduce sexual interest, as may the side effects from medications taken for, say, the treatment of depressive disorders or blood pressure control. Illness or apathy of the partner, hot flushes and sleep disturbance can also reduce sexual interest and desire.

Sexual problems may stem from longstanding dissatisfaction or disappointment that over the years sexual fulfilment has not been achieved; poor communication and lack of warmth and closeness in sexual relationships may be responsible. Erection problems in the partner may have occurred before the female menopause, producing resentment and sadness. Difficulties such as these are common in men over 50 years of age but can be effectively treated in some cases by counselling, or by penile prosthetic surgery or injections self-administered by the male partner to produce erection enhancement.

Impotence in the male is sometimes related to the female menopause. In this case it usually stems from fear of hurting the partner, and may be compounded by a lack of arousal in the woman.

Poor penile erection, with consequent short erection time, may lead to a feeling of frustration on both sides and increasing loss of interest by the woman.

Sexual disorders may include painful intercourse (dyspareunia), lack of orgasm – often due to loss in quality of pleasurable genital sensation – and reduced arousal. Oestrogen therapy is of benefit here, and the application of a lubricant (see page 93) can ease discomfort and heighten tactile sensation.

It is true that sexual function may be reduced as the result of menopausal symptoms such as tiredness, irritability and depression. Conflicts arising from sexual difficulties tend to magnify sexual problems and further reduce sexual desire.

In Western society attitudes towards sex have changed greatly over the last few decades. The use of the oral contraceptive pill has been partly responsible, but greater freedom and openness in the discussion of sexual matters have been of equal importance. Today women should expect continuation of a healthy sex life far beyond the menopause. The understanding and communication of problems will help them to achieve, and sustain, a fulfilling sex life.

CHAPTER 3

OSTEOPOROSIS

TWO particular disorders are associated with the peri-menopause and beyond: osteoporosis and cardiovascular disease. Both can be prevented, or significantly reduced in their effects, by a healthy lifestyle and appropriate therapy.

Bone structure

Bones are designed to withstand the amount of stress and strain the body imposes on them. Those that will take more stress are denser and more compact. Bone has an outer sheath or membrane called the periosteum covering the dense outer compact bone (the **cortical layer**). Below this is the spongy or **trabecular layer** of bone.

Within the leg and arm bones, which contain little trabecular substance except at their ends, are hollow spaces filled with bone marrow. The wrist bones, the vertebrae and the neck of the femur contain not bone marrow space but trabecular bone. Vertebrae have little of the heavy cortical bone, but their cubical shape lends strength to their trabecular composition.

Bone formation

Bone is a connective tissue which reaches its peak of density around the age of 35. It is made up of approximately one-third collagen (the **matrix**) and two-thirds **mineral**.

The protein collagen, along with the protein elastin and a further, fibrous protein called GAGS, contributes strength to bone by means of its scaffolding. Collagen greatly increases the elastic properties of

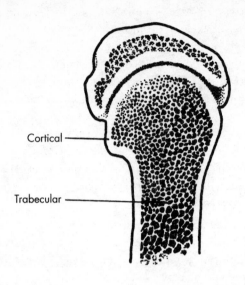

Cortical

Trabecular

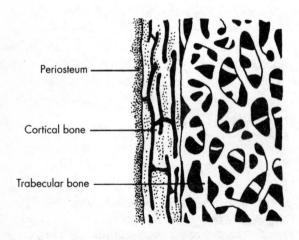

Periosteum

Cortical bone

Trabecular bone

Figure 5   Structure of long bone

bone and helps to prevent stretching forces. GAGS increase turgidity and resist compressive forces. The mineral component of bone is mainly calcium, and when this is lost the bone becomes brittle.

Bone is constantly 'remodelling' itself by the action of **osteoblast** cells, which lay down the matrix and help to deposit calcium, and **osteoclast** cells (originating from bone marrow), which destroy collagen and break down, or resorb, bone. Through a complicated process called 'coupling' osteoclast cells can form young osteoblasts, setting in motion the remodelling process. Osteoclasts and osteoblasts are therefore responsible for both the resorption and the laying down of bone. Their action is controlled, negatively and positively, by bone-active hormones and growth factors. These are:

parathyroid hormone (PTH)	– acts on osteoblasts
calcitonin	– acts on osteoclasts
vitamin D3	– acts on osteoclasts and osteoblasts
insulin	– promotes growth of bone cells
oestrogen	– acts on osteoblasts
progesterone	– acts on osteoblasts.

Oestrogen prevents resorption of bone, and progesterone promotes its formation by locking on to osteoblast cells. Studies also show that the lowered levels of both oestrogen and progesterone resulting from irregular ovulation in the peri-menopausal years and post-menopausal lack of ovulation influence bone loss. It is becoming clearer that progesterone plays a very important role in bone remodelling through its influence on the 'coupling' process. Post-menopausal osteoporosis is in part, therefore, a progesterone-deficiency disease.

Osteoporosis

As a result of ovarian failure and higher-than-normal excretion of bone calcium in the urine, collagen and mineral levels fall and bone mass is reduced: this condition is known as osteoporosis. The normal ageing process produces Type II osteoporosis, whereas Type I results from premature ovarian failure. Type II is seen in both men and women over the age of 60 and is probably more directly responsible for fractures of the femur in older women than Type I. The two types of osteoporosis represent different bone-loss processes, which

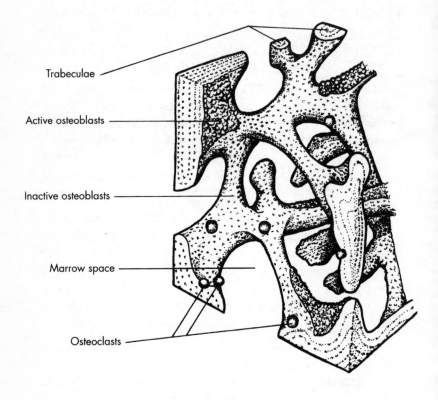

Trabeculae

Active osteoblasts

Inactive osteoblasts

Marrow space

Osteoclasts

Figure 6   Structure of trabecular bone

merge in later life to cause susceptibility to fractures, loss of height and deformity of the spine.

Any condition which causes menstruation to stop (amenorrhoea) will upset ovulation, with consequent reduction in the availability of oestrogen and progesterone. The likelihood of premature osteoporosis developing is increased by the following: Turner's syndrome (a congenital failure of the ovaries to develop); amenorrhoea caused by too much prolactin in the blood; amenorrhoea caused by excessive physical exercise; amenorrhoea caused by anorexia nervosa; and amenorrhoea caused by drugs used in the treatment of endometriosis and polycystic ovarian syndrome. 'Athletic amenorrhea' is becoming more common with the increasing popularity among women for marathons and other endurance activities. The restricted diet and intense training may also play a part in reducing body fat and psychological stress. As many as half of the top-class female runners, rowers, cyclists and ballet dancers are known to be amenorrhoeic.

Regular weight-bearing exercise in moderation – say, for 20-30 minutes three or four times a week – will help protect bones from loss of density. In the younger woman repetitive weight-bearing exercise, such as running/jogging, tennis, basketball, volleyball, brisk walking and aerobic dance is most beneficial. In older women walking is most beneficial in reducing the risk of osteoporosis, but exercise alone is not as effective as oestrogen replacement. Muscle tone and balance will be improved and hence the risk of fractures caused by falls will be reduced.

Each year, about 40 per cent of trabecular bone and 10 per cent of cortical bone are remodelled. Over an average lifetime a woman may lose about 25-35 per cent of her cortical bone (mainly from the arms and legs), and about 40-50 per cent of trabecular bone. Men, who continue to produce the protective male hormone androgen, lose only two-thirds of this amount.

In women, trabecular bone loss starts as early as 35. The loss (mainly from the vertebrae, wrists and lower jaw) is slow at first, but by the time the menopause is reached constitutes 3-5 per cent per year. This rate persists for another 5-10 years, then slows. Cortical bone loss starts about 10 years later, and is equal in both sexes at the age of 45. In women, the rate is 2-3 per cent per year in the 5-10 years after menopause, then slows.

The amount of bone loss varies from person to person. The reasons for this are uncertain, but factors that are known to influence it are premature menopause (natural or surgical) before the age of 45; osteoporosis in a close female relative; high alcohol intake; cigarette-smoking; low body mass – i.e. small stature and small bones; inadequate calcium intake in youth; no pregnancies; existing disease of the bones; sedentary lifestyle; long-term use of cortico-steroid drugs or thyroxine; anorexia nervosa; caffeine; steroids for arthritis, asthma or ulcerative colitis; and some drugs used in the treatment of epilepsy and endometriosis. It is known that Asian and Caucasian women are more prone to bone loss than women of African origin.

The prevalence and cost of bone fracture

Women (of all ages) sustain 50-70 fractures per 1,000 per year, a rate 8-10 times higher than that in men. Fifty per cent of women will sustain a significant osteoporotic fracture during their lifetime. Vertebral fractures can cause collapse or wedging of the bones, resulting in a bent back and a 'dowager's hump'. Loss of height occurs, accompanied by either high or low back pain depending upon the site of collapse.

The associated death rate, from pneumonia, blood clots, infection, stroke and so on, can be as high as 50 per cent within the year following a hip fracture. Only 25-50 per cent of women who survive after sustaining this type of fracture ever regain their full pre-fracture level of function.

In England and Wales in excess of 60,000 hip fractures occur annually, costing the taxpayer £220 million, and this is rising dramatically. About 7 per cent of women and 3 per cent of men sustain a fracture of the forearm, vertebrae or femur by the age of 60, and this rises to 25 per cent and 8 per cent respectively by the 80th birthday.

In the USA 500,000 vertebral fractures and 200,000 hip fractures occur each year. The remainder of the 1.5 million new fractures are of the wrist, shoulder, pelvis and ankle. Fifty per cent of the total are the result of osteoporosis. Fracture treatment costs a staggering US$18 billion overall. As the number of elderly grow both in the USA and the UK, such costs can only rise further.

Predicting osteoporosis and bone fracture

Apart from the predisposing factors listed on page 45, fracture risk can be predicted by identifying those with reduced bone mineral content or bone density. An early fracture before the menopause, or even before 60, is likely to increase the risk of fracture at a related site later in life. Studies are taking place to investigate the possible relationship between skin thickness and bone mass, which could indicate. that estimating skin thickness is an effective way to screen women at risk of developing osteoporosis. There is also a new blood test that can identify women at risk by pinpointing changes on the vitamin D receptor gene. The test needs modifying before general introduction.

Recently developed screening techniques have made it possible to measure bone density. Such screening is expensive, but could in future help to cut the costs of fracture treatment.

Of the four available methods, dual absorptiometry (DPA) is useful for lumbar spine and hip bone mineral measurement. Accuracy is within 3-6 per cent for the spine, and 3-4 per cent for the hip. Radiation exposure is low.

Quantitative computed tomography (QCT) is less precise, more expensive and requires greater radiation exposure than DPA.

Single photon absorptiometry (SPA) is convenient for measurement of the forearm site. Accuracy is within 4-5 per cent and radiation exposure low. SPA may be cheaper for mass screening, but the result may be misleading with regard to comparative changes in the bones of other areas, such as the spine or hips.

Dual energy X-ray absorptiometry (DEXA) represents the most recent technological advance. The time required to scan the spine is only seven minutes, compared to 20 minutes for DPA, which reduces radiation exposure. Accuracy and precision are excellent, within 0.5-1.2 per cent. An X-ray beam of approximately 6 mm is used to scan the site, and a detector on the opposite side of the patient decodes the information.

The diagnosis of osteoporosis and prediction of fracture risk by such techniques are the most accurate currently available. The combination of one measurement of bone mass in the forearm along with new biochemical markers of bone formation (for example, osteocalcin) may be able, in future, reliably to identify at the menopause those women who are at greatest risk of developing osteoporosis in 10-12 years' time.

The cost of screening has to be carefully weighed against the cost of treating the rising number of osteoporosis sufferers, currently estimated at 2,000,000 in the UK. The increasing cost to the nation of osteoporosis followed by fracture and fracture complication would seem to favour the phasing-in of a screening programme, perhaps giving priority in the first instance to those most at risk (see page 46). Further studies are required before the value of bone density measurements in such a programme can be assessed.

Treatment for osteoporosis

Prevention is the most cost-effective approach and should start in childhood. It requires a well-balanced diet rich in calcium and adequate vitamin D; not smoking, and moderating alcohol intake (both produce toxins that inhibit the beneficial effect of ovarian hormones); and steady, regular weight-bearing exercise. Observing these recommendations will help women to acquire a maximal bone density which can persist throughout adult life.

The use of HRT for the prevention of osteoporosis is discussed in Chapter 5. It is very effective in preventing bone loss when taken at and after the menopause and its effects last even if HRT is taken ten or more years after the menopause. It is also safe and effective even if started and continued more than 15 years after the menopause.

For women who do not wish to take sex hormone therapy, or who have been advised against it on medical grounds, there are other treatments to combat bone loss:

Etidronate This is a bisphosphonate. It is taken on a 90-day cycle: 400 mg etidronate disodium daily for the first 14 days followed by a 500 mg calcium supplement for the next 76 days. The cycle is repeated and continued for a recommended three years. Etidronate (Didronel) is taken with water or fruit juice on an empty stomach two hours before or after food. This cyclical, non-hormonal treatment is used only for osteoporosis of the spine: it does not prevent it, nor is it a painkiller.

Newer, more powerful, bisphosphonates are being researched.

In severe cases of osteoporosis both HRT and Didronel are safe if prescribed together, but no research is available to establish any added benefit from using both.

Calcitonin This hormone is produced by the thyroid gland of certain fish. it hinders the action of cells which break down bone and hence improves bone mass. As well as preventing osteoporosis it is an effective painkiller. It is usually restricted to use in hospitals, where it is injected by a specialist.

Another form of it is salcatonin, derived from salmon. New forms, either available now or being developed, are nasal sprays and suppositories.

The importance of calcium and vitamin D are discussed in Chapter 7.

New treatments, and those under research, include raloxifene, ipriflavone, parathyroid hormone, and fluoride in association with calcium supplementation.

CHAPTER 4

CARDIOVASCULAR DISEASE

THE BRITISH ISLES and the Scandinavian countries have the highest incidence of cardiovascular disease in the world. Women in Great Britain are more likely to die from coronary heart disease than from any other medical problem.[1] Complications arising in the cardiovascular system are responsible for a quarter of a million deaths annually in the USA. The fact that women experience anginal-type chest pain more commonly than men (56 per cent as against 43 per cent) and currently outnumber men in the occurrence of coronary death is largely related to the fact that women live longer.[2] Evidence of heart disease in women usually starts to become evident as coronary heart disease ten years later than in men.[4] Before the Framingham Heart Study[3] was first published, in the USA in the early 1970s, physicians relied for prevention and management of coronary heart disease on studies based upon observations of middle-aged men. The Framingham study, however, was misleading as it suggested that one male in four who had angina would incur a heart attack (myocardial infarction) within the next five years, whereas 86 per cent of women who had angina would not. Angina, therefore, was wrongly perceived as a benign (unimportant) problem in women.[5]

It was only after publication of the Coronary Artery Surgery Study[6] that it became quite clear that, after coronary artery evaluation using the technique of arteriography to define better the size of the coronary arteries, angina in women between the ages of 60 and 69 had the same poor outlook – that is, progression to heart attack – as in the men in the Framingham Study.

There is a gender difference in the occurrence of heart attack between men and women, 38 and 50 per cent respectively, but once a heart attack occurs there is higher fatality in women compared to men, 39 per cent *versus* 31 per cent.[7]

Angina and myocardial infarction management for men and women

Reports show that women with chest pain, or established heart disease, are subjected to fewer invasive diagnostic and other procedures than men: whether the difference is appropriate or inappropriate may be revealed by further reports.

It is possible that this difference in evaluation may be due to physician or patient decisions, or to family pressures on patients, or indeed to elderly women relying upon family and friends to make decisions for them.[8]

Exercise electrocardiograms in older women often give an inadequate result owing to associated illness, excess weight, elevated blood pressure, and so on. Exercise testing using the drug Thallium gives a more accurate assessment, but initially it was only used in men because early testing in women gave false positive results until it was realised that the breasts distorted the analyses of the result due to defects in the 'perfusion process'.[10,11] Now the predictive value of the test has been improved and is useful. Usually if the Thallium exercise test result is abnormal the patient will be advised to proceed to the more accurate test of coronary arteriography. Coronary arteriography is the next step to a heart revascularisation procedure (that is, angioplasty or bypass surgery). It is interesting that in the USA in 1987 an extensive study showed that ten times more men than women were referred for coronary arteriography following an abnormal Thallium exercise test, yet anti-anginal medication was prescribed equally for both sexes.[9,12,16]

Investigation of drug therapy used for the treatment of angina and the further prevention of heart attacks shows that few have undergone random gender comparison testing, which is essential to determine preference both in performance and dosage for women compared to men. The timolol maleate trial[13] in Europe is an exception. This B-blocker (Betim) showed equal benefit to both sexes in both short- and long-term use. Aspirin in the ISIS-2 trial also confirmed equal gender benefit.[14] Other drugs frequently used in the treatment of angina and following a heart attack (myocardial infarction) have not undergone sufficient gender comparison.

Following a heart attack fewer women than men are referred by their physician or cardiologist for exercise rehabilitation, despite the evidence that equal benefit for both sexes results from exercise training and fitness advice.[15]

During the 1980s the poor evaluation of Thallium scanning diminished confidence in exercise diagnostic testing for heart disease in women. Now, however, interpretation has improved and positron emission tomography (PET) and echo-cardiography are in use.[17, 18] More accurate information about heart disease in both sexes can now be obtained and coronary arteriography can be carried out as the next step for those affected who warrant this procedure.

The continuing problem, however, is that cardiac revascularisation (bypass surgery) risk remains twice as high in women as it is in men. The record of increased death rate in women is confined to the hospital stay period. Women who do survive to be discharged have five to ten further years of comparable or better life quality than men.

Care of the female heart

Prevention of heart disease begins with sensible exercise, a balanced diet which will also control weight, a low alcohol intake and not smoking (as discussed later in this chapter and in other chapters).

Good medical and surgical care following a heart attack and bypass surgery will enhance survival. Early detection of diabetes mellitus, hypertension and obesity will reduce the incidence of coronary heart disease. In those who do develop it, early diagnosis will reduce the need for bypass surgery in older women, for whom the post-operative risk is greater. The use of HRT at the menopause and beyond can reduce cardiovascular disease by approximatley 40 per cent.[19]

The risk of developing cardiovascular disease is greater for those to whom any of the following apply: premature menopause; hereditary hypercholesterolaemia (an inherited high level of cholesterol in the blood); a family history of coronary heart disease; hypertension; diabetes; cigarette-smoking; obesity; an achievement-orientated, competitive personality ('Type A' – see page 112); a sedentary lifestyle; and a diet high in saturated fat and low in fruit, vegetables, starch and fibre.

Worldwide, coronary heart disease is six times lower in women than in men between the ages of 35 and 44, but only two times lower by the age of 50. At 75 and beyond its incidence is the same in both sexes. The reason would appear to stem, in part, from the changes which occur in women around the menopause in the arteries and blood factors. Blood factors which rise at this time, when oestrogen levels drop, are fibrinogen and factor VIIc (which increase clotting). The anti-clotting agent antithrombin III falls. Blood cholesterol also rises. The fact that coronary heart disease is much higher in women who undergo a premature menopause before the age of 40 lends weight to the theory that coronary heart disease risk is increased by menopausal changes.[21, 22]

Numerous and extensive studies have concluded that the ovarian sex hormones give protection against coronary heart disease. It is also possible that rising levels of follicle-stimulating hormone from the pituitary gland, along with other hormone-like substances such as prostaglandins, may have an indirect adverse effect on blood fats, on the size of blood vessels, and on blood–clotting processes.[22, 23, 24]

Oestrogen and heart disease

Since a Mayo Clinic study 40 years ago showed that women who have had both ovaries removed develop severe coronary artery narrowing as frequently as men of similar age, it has been suggested that oestrogen can help prevent heart disease.

The ability of oestrogen to protect the arteries, confirmed in recent studies, arises from its beneficial effect on blood fats (lipids).

There is also evidence that oestrogen has a direct effect on blood vessel walls. The lining cells of blood vessels (endothelium) respond directly through oestrogen receptors in the cell and dilate. This allows more blood to flow, resulting in an increase of oxygen supply to the heart muscle, and helps to protect against angina and blood clotting, which are associated with narrowing of the coronary arteries.[25, 26]

A recent study in *The Lancet* confirms the protective effect of oestrogen on the artery endothelial lining, but also suggests that oestrogen acts directly on the smooth muscle of the artery itself producing a relaxing, widening action and an improved blood flow. Probably 70-80 per cent of the beneficial effect of HRT on cardiovascular risk is not produced by improvement in blood fat levels but is a direct effect of oestrogen on the arterial blood vessel wall.[27, 28]

Cerebrovascular disease

Women of 50 and over have a 20 per cent chance of having a stroke and an 8 per cent chance that the stroke will be fatal. A stroke is caused by either a blood clot or a haemorrhage in the brain, usually related to blood pressure, smoking, or fatty deposits lining the arteries of the body.

A link has been established between certain types of oestrogen and stroke, but stroke is more likely to be related to blood fat (lipoprotein) changes. Lipoprotein changes, however, have little relationship to cerebrovascular disease in comparison to their effect on coronary heart disease.[29]

Blood fats

Blood fats, or lipids, come in various forms. These include cholesterol, triglycerides and free fatty acids. Cholesterol is found in all body tissues as well as in hormones. The amount of cholesterol in the blood is dependent upon factors such as age, sex, diet, heredity and lifestyle. Cholesterol exists in many forms: very low-, low- and high-density, along with other sub-groups.

Cholesterol is transported in the bloodstream by lipoproteins. High-density cholesterol (HDL) is taken to the liver for breakdown and the low-density form (LDL) to organs and tissues for their use. The LDLs tend to stick to the walls of arteries, but the HDLs and their important sub-group HDL_2 do not. The very low-density lipoproteins (VLDL) carry a type of fat called triglyceride. They are formed of glycerol and three fatty acids, and are linked to coronary heart disease because of their influence on blood clotting.

Before the menopause, women show higher levels of the protective HDL and HDL_2 cholesterol, but a lower level of the harmful LDL cholesterol than do men. (Ideally, the protective HDL should be at or above 23 per cent of the total cholesterol figure.)

HDL lessens the risk of coronary heart disease and is influenced by the circulating blood levels of oestrogen and progesterone. The latter causes the triglyceride levels to be kept low, thereby reducing the risk of blood clotting.

Women after the menopause have a high risk of coronary heart disease. Oestrogen administration can reduce this risk substantially through its action of increasing the protective HDL cholesterol and reducing the damaging LDL cholesterol. A commonly prescribed oral oestrogen with progestogen (Prempak-C) and an oestrogen used as a 'patch' with progestogen (Estracombi) are shown to lower total cholesterol and LDL cholesterol in much the same way, increasing the protective HDL cholesterol. [30]

Every 1 mg/dl increase in blood level HDL is associated with a decrease of approximately 3-5 per cent in the risk of coronary heart disease.

Every 1 mg/dl decrease in harmful LDL is associated with a decline of approximately 2 per cent in the risk of coronary heart disease. Changes caused by oestrogen can lead, therefore, to a relatively large decrease in risk. [31]

Evaluation of commonly known blood fats suggests that other lipoproteins may be of greater importance in terms of causing cardiovascular risk. An example is lipoprotein (a), or Lp(a). High levels are associated with a higher risk of coronary heart disease. A recent study confirms that there is a direct relationship between a woman's age and Lp(a) levels. Oestrogen deficiency or reduction influences Lp(a) production in the body. At age 50-55 levels of Lp(a) rise from an average pre-menopause level of 9.6 mg/dl to a post-menopausal average of 15.1 mg/dl. The use of HRT (oestrogen and progestogen) can improve not only the Lp(a) level, but raise the protective HDL cholesterol and lower the harmful LDL cholesterol. [32, 33, 34]

Users of HRT are at half the risk from cardiovascular disease as compared to non-users.

The distribution of body fat can signal blood fat changes and a greater or lesser risk of developing coronary heart disease. Android (male) fat distribution over the upper body and abdominal wall, in particular, signals adverse blood fat profile, and a rise in the level of insulin in the blood. Gynoid (female) fat distribution over the hips and thighs appears to carry no significant risk for coronary heart disease. If HRT is taken after the menopause android fat, as compared to gynoid fat, will reduce, with an associated improvement in the blood lipid levels generally.[35, 36]

Blood clotting

Fatty deposits (atheromatous plaques) on the walls of the arteries, caused in part by increased LDL blood levels, assist in forming the plaques to which sticky cells (platelets) in the blood adhere, and with the addition of fibrin, a protein that promotes clotting, trigger the occurrence of a blood clot (thrombosis). The actions of fibrinogen, thrombin and factors VIIc, X and XII also contribute to the clotting processes.

Antithrombin III helps combat the clotting effect of thrombin. There is also a method by which the body can dissolve fibrin, thereby reducing platelet activity and the risk of thrombosis. These latter protective mechanisms seem to be set at a higher level in women than in men, *but only before the menopause*. This also holds true for the increase in the protective HDL and HDL_2 observed in women before the menopause.

The Northwick Park Heart Study, published in *The Lancet* in 1983, reported significant increases in both clotting factors and cholesterol in women undergoing a natural menopause. There were also changes in fibrinogen levels and cholesterol in a smaller number of women studied who had undergone an artificial menopause. These findings support the view that oestrogen helps to combat the development of cardiovascular disease.

In summary, therefore, there is an increased risk of coronary heart disease at and after the menopause. What is not entirely clear, however, is whether reduced oestrogen is entirely responsible for the lipid and blood–clotting changes that are likely to take place around this time. Other factors such as the rising follicle-stimulating hormone level, the influences of prostaglandins, nutrition, exercise, lifestyle and the individual's response to stress no doubt also play a part in this complex process.

The insulin factor

Numerous risk factors for cardiovascular disease, including obesity, hypertension, adverse lipid changes, diabetes, changes in coagulation (blood clotting and fibrinogen) and reduced sex hormones at the menopause, have been the subject of discussion. These are all inter-related.

As a woman ages the body becomes less responsive to insulin produced by the pancreas and the insulin level rises. Consequently the control of carbohydrate breakdown in food and blood sugar is less well managed. Oestrogen tends to restore normal insulin and blood sugar levels.

Research suggests that the disturbance of insulin and sugar balance at the menopause may be the pivotal linking mechanism for developing cardiovascular disease risk at this stage in life.[37, 38, 39]

CHAPTER 5

MANAGING THE MENOPAUSE WITH HORMONE REPLACEMENT THERAPY

DURING the peri-menopause and beyond, the lack of the hormones oestrogen and progesterone and subsequent changes in body chemicals are likely to bring about physical and emotional disruption. The belief that if periods start early the menopause will be early and, correspondingly, a late start indicates a late menopause is incorrect. Many women follow the pattern of their mothers, but the onset of the natural menopause can never be predicted.

The symptoms a woman experiences at this time of life may not be the same in degree as those perceived by her mother, sister or girlfriend. Everyone is different, and hormones and other factors affect people in a variety of ways. The hormone concentration in the bloodstream bears no relation to the severity or otherwise of menopausal symptoms. Not all women will have all the typical symptoms of the menopause, and some women find that one symptom predominates over the others.

How the menopause is managed depends on individual needs – but successful management depends on a woman's awareness of the changes taking place in her body. Finding out about the menopause will make her better equipped for discussion with her doctor concerning the most acceptable management regimen. Ideally, discussion should start before menopausal symptoms begin, and whether she decides to take hormone replacement therapy or not, it will still be helpful for her to follow the guidelines for healthy nutrition, exercise and stress management described in Chapter 7.

Choosing a doctor

Some doctors hold set opinions concerning treatment regimens for the menopause, and some may be unwilling to devote time to counselling. Evidence shows that too many women leave the consulting room with a prescription for a sedative or tranquilliser when what they really wanted was clear advice on what to do.

If you feel your own doctor is not sympathetic to your problems, that you are being rushed or communication is poor, you may ask to be referred to a gynaecologist or a special menopause clinic. In the UK such clinics are often attached to NHS teaching hospitals. Alternatively, you could see a gynaecologist privately or attend one of the many private 'well woman' clinics (see 'Useful addresses'). In Canada and the USA no referral is required.

Some methods of alleviating menopausal symptoms can be employed without medical advice; others, such as hormone replacement therapy, require discussion with a doctor. The pros and cons of the latter options are reviewed here.

Hormone replacement therapy (HRT)

In North America 3,500 women each day experience the menopause, the cessation of menstrual periods, and within the next decade 50 million women will be post-menopausal. Complaints associated with menopausal symptoms have been estimated to initiate about 1 million visits to the doctor each year in Canada, 70 per cent of these to the general practitioner. In the USA and Canada, where it is vigorously promoted to the public, about 80 per cent of women with menopausal symptoms receive HRT. In the UK about 20 per cent, or one woman in five, receives HRT. The number of post-menopausal women will have reached 14 million by the year 2000, when one woman in three is likely to receive HRT. Attitudes to health care, as well as the socio-economic climate of these countries, are different, but perhaps more important is the conservatism – some might say scepticism – of the UK in relation to new approaches and treatments. Nevertheless, Britain is in the forefront of menopausal research, especially with regard to safe hormone therapy techniques.

HRT (oestrogen alone, without progesterone) was first used in the 1950s for control of hot flushes, sweats, vaginal dryness, joint discomfort and urinary problems. The following 20 years showed that women who took HRT also had less osteoporosis and suffered fewer heart attacks and strokes. It became apparent that HRT given at this time in a woman's life had significant preventive value as well as providing the immediate benefit of symptom relief.

By the 1960s it had become clear that if the uterus was still present oestrogen alone was not enough. A synthetic progesterone drug, called a progestogen, had to be added to the monthly oestrogen regimen to protect against the thickening effect (hyperplasia) caused by oestrogen on the endometrium, or lining of the uterus. The duration of progestogen use rather than the dosage is more important in the prevention of hyperplasia, which can lead to endometrial cancer. Oestrogen given alone (unopposed therapy) is associated with a 7-15 per cent increased risk of hyperplasia. When progestogen is added for seven days each month (opposed therapy), the risk of hyperplasia is reduced to 5 per cent, and to zero if the course lasts 12-13 days in each cycle.

Since the 1960s great advances have been made in the way HRT can be used as well as in its safety.

When to start HRT

A considerable reduction in ovarian sex hormones occurs about two to three years before menstruation finally stops. Significant bone loss can occur during this transition phase, when infrequent periods and other peri-menopausal symptoms such as hot flushes, sweats and dryness of the vagina are experienced. If these vasomotor symptoms are mild, simple self-help measures and a non-hormone approach as suggested in Chapter 7 may be sufficient.

If the symptoms become severe and disruptive the commencement of HRT could be considered at this time, especially if menstruation is becoming infrequent. The preventive effect for osteoporosis and coronary heart disease will be an important bonus. Hot flushes, sweats and vaginal dryness will be greatly alleviated within 7-10 days of starting HRT.

Some women, however (perhaps up to 15 per cent), find they are intolerant of HRT; they tend to experience symptoms such as fluid retention, breast tenderness, weight gain, nausea, headaches, itching skin and rashes, and PMS-type symptoms.

Women who have had a premature menopause or surgical removal of the ovaries (oöphorectomy) will be advised by their doctors to start HRT (provided there are no health factors that make it inadvisable). It will immediately help to control menopausal symptoms as well as providing long-term preventive benefits.

There appears to be no age above which HRT should not be considered, but if opposed therapy provokes recommencement of vaginal bleeding, where the uterus is still present, this may not be acceptable to a woman who is many years past the menopause. Breast tenderness is also more likely to occur in this context, and research has not yet clarified whether the protective effect on bone and blood vessels is as great.

Another (controversial) form of therapy for certain cases in the over-70 age group where osteoporosis is very troublesome, causing pain and extreme weakness, is the use of an anabolic steroid (stanazolol); this can improve the quality of life and retard osteoporosis, but may provoke menstrual bleeding.

There is plenty of evidence to suggest that HRT benefits elderly women with osteoporosis, preventing further bone loss and even to some degree reversing it. If oestrogen/progestogen combinations are used, the oestrogen-induced breast tenderness which is commonly experienced may be overcome by starting the oestrogen (in combined therapy) at a very low dose, then increasing it gradually after 4-6 weeks to the more appropriate bone-protective level.

Whatever the patient's age, HRT is of course more likely to prove successful with considerate counselling and careful clinical management.

When to stop HRT

Most women who start HRT do so to reduce peri-menopausal symptoms because these have become troublesome and affect their daily living; others take it because they have experienced premature menopause, have had hysterectomies with removal of the ovaries or are at risk of osteoporosis. There is at present no consensus as to how long HRT should continue for optimal long-term benefit. Treatment for three to five years is usually sufficient to relieve annoying symptoms, but for the protection of bones and blood vessels therapy should continue for much longer.

If HRT is carefully managed, as detailed later in this chapter, and the risk/benefit ratio is closely monitored, there is no reason why it should not be continued for 20 years or more. HRT should not be stopped suddenly but discontinued gradually over several months to reduce the possibility of symptoms recurring.

Types of HRT

HRT preparations may be administered by mouth, as a skin gel, as a skin patch, as an implant or by vaginal creams and pessaries.

Oestrogens can be either natural or synthetic. Natural oestrogens are of animal origin, the commonest source being pregnant mares. These animals supply oestrogen in the form of **equilin** and **equilenin.** The equilin, in the form of sodium equilin sulphate, is paired (conjugated) with sodium oestrone sulphate to produce the commonly prescribed preparation Premarin.

Synthetic oestrogens are chemically dissimilar to their natural cousins and tend to have a more profound effect on the liver proteins, producing greater changes in blood clotting and blood lipid levels. Such products, for example **ethinyl oestradiol,** should therefore not be used for HRT.

Oral therapy

This is at present the commonest method of administration in the US and UK. By this means the hormone is taken, immediately after absorption, into the bloodstream and then to the liver, where up to one-third is converted to the less potent oestrone and oestriol. Higher doses consequently need to be given to achieve a satisfactory therapeutic blood **oestradiol** level. Nausea is often reported by those who take HRT by mouth.

The higher doses required by this method of administration can also influence liver metabolism, producing a rise in the sex hormone binding globulin, a sensitive indicator of liver protein function. Changes in triglyceride levels, with a rise in the VLDLs and a decrease in the antithrombin blood-clotting factor, may occur. These changes, which are dose-related, are seen when oral oestrogen is used in either the 17B-oestradiol form or the conjugated equine variety, but are more likely to occur with the latter.

Skin patch

When 17B-oestradiol, the natural oestrogen closest to human oestrogen, is administered transdermally, or by skin patch, nausea is rare, and the passage of the drug through the liver is avoided. There are no changes in the sex hormone binding globulin, or to the blood lipids or clotting factors. The skin patch was introduced to the UK in the mid-1980s under the brand name Estraderm. It consists of four layers: an outer transparent layer, a drug reservoir, a polymer membrane, and an adhesive outer rim. A continuous controlled amount of 17B-oestradiol is delivered through the skin at a rate sufficient to produce pre-menopausal blood oestradiol levels. The patch, which comes in three strengths (25, 50 and 100 micrograms, indicating relative absorption within a 24-hour period), needs changing every three to four days.

About 5 per cent of skin patch users report skin irritation and itching at the site of application, caused by the adhesive rim on the patch disc, not the drug. Another 5 per cent find that the patch loosens at the edges before it is time to change it, while approximately 10 per cent of users report difficulty in taking the disc off its backing prior to application.

A new form of delivering 17B-oestradiol by skin patch, Evorel, is less likely, owing to its construction, to cause irritation and itching. It is also easier to remove from its backing.

A current drawback of this patch is that only one dosage form is available, at 50 micrograms. A Swiss study confirms that Evorel provides the same protection against post-menopausal bone loss as taking 2 mg daily of oral micronised oestradiol valerate (Climaval or Progynova).

Implants

Subcutaneous implants of 17B-oestradiol were first used in the 1960s. Now perfected, they are offered by many clinics, especially in the UK. This method of delivery also avoids the passage of the oestrogen through the liver. Implants last from three to six months, the reappearance of menopausal symptoms indicating when another implant is required. The implant, about the size of a small pea, is inserted in the fatty tissue below the skin surface of the abdominal wall or the thigh, under local skin anaesthetic. The small pellet, 25, 50 or 100 mg in strength, releases a continuous supply of oestradiol.

Using the patch

Even when using a sticking paster, applying it correctly can make a big difference to how well it sticks. This also applies to your patch treatment. The hints and tips that follow should help to ensure that your patches stick well.

Removing the protective backing

The protective backing can be removed easily in one of the two ways shown in the illustrations. Do not touch the sticky surface of the patch with your fingers or allow the patch to become wrinkled so that the sticky surfaces come into contact with each other.

Method 1(a) Method 1(b) Method 2

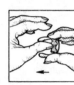 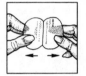

Bend the patch.   Pull patch with
your thumb.
Push away
backing.

Remove the
backing.

Site of application

Apply to a flat, non-hairy area where skin does not crease and clothes are not likely to catch. The buttocks are often the best areas but other places can be used. Find the best area for you by trying different places, e.g. thighs, lower back and so on. Do *not* apply to the breasts.

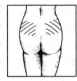

The skin

Make sure the skin is clean and dry. Water or sweat on the skin may stop the patch sticking properly. Wait for at least 15 minutes after a bath or shower before applying the patch, as skin can still be slightly moist after towel-drying. Avoid using bath oil or greasy lotion, as these leave a film on the skin that can stop the patch sticking properly.

Pressure
The adhesive is sensitive to pressure and warmth. To ensure the patch sticks well it is very important to press it in place with the flat of the hand for at least 10 seconds. Then run your fingers round the edge of the patch to seal it in position.

Will the patches re-stick more than once?

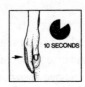

Your patch can be re-stuck if it comes off, or if you take it off for a long, hot bath, a sauna or sunbed session. Re-apply exactly as you would a new patch. Normally each patch can be removed and re-applied once or twice before losing its stickiness.

Do not remove a patch soon after putting it on as the glue tends to be soft when first exposed. Taking it off too soon can leave the soft glue on your skin rather than on the patch.

Can I wear my patch in the bath and to swim?
If you have a long, hot bath, the patch may not stick so well. To avoid this, remove the patch beforehand and keep it on a dry piece of plastic or foil whilst you are in the bath. Re-apply once your skin is completely dry again (15 minutes).

What should I do if a patch comes off?
In the unlikely event that a patch falls off, you can re-apply it in the same way as you would a new patch. If it comes off while you are in the bath or shower, pick it up by its edge, shake the water off and re-apply when your skin is completely dry.

Won't the patch come off during the night?
This should not happen, but a patch could be pulled off if a loose edge is caught by a nightdress or bedding, so before going to sleep just check that the edges of the patch are well stuck down.

Can I have a sauna or use a sunbed?
Always cover the patch with your swimsuit before sunbathing. Skin becomes very moist in a sauna or on a sunbed and this may cause the patch to stick less well. When applying a patch after sauna or sunbed treatment, remember that your skin will remain moist for some time afterwards. Wait until it is properly dry before applying a patch. Try to plan saunas or sunbed treatments for the days when you change your patch. If you like to have saunas or sunbed sessions more than twice a week, you may need to remove your patch and re-apply afterwards (keep the sachet and protective backing for storing the patch).

Why would a patch come off two days after sticking very well?
This can happen if you have oily skin. Your skin produces oil over two days which can stop the patch sticking. It may also become detached if your skin is very dry and peeling (e.g. after sunbathing). In such cases, try to find an area where your skin is not oily or has not been exposed to the sun.

Occasionally a small quantity of the male hormone testosterone is combined with the oestradiol to increase sexual drive in cases where reduced libido is a significant problem at the menopause. (Testosterone should not be taken by mouth as it may adversely affect the liver.)

Major swings in the blood oestradiol level can occur with implant usage. Menopausal symptoms may reappear when oestradiol blood levels are normal: this occurrence is called 'tachyphylaxis' and may indicate either poor absorption of the oestradiol in the areas where it is taken up, or a developing dependency on oestradiol itself, though there is no evidence of oestradiol addiction. Careful and frequent monitoring of blood oestradiol levels is required so that a level of about 250 pico mols per litre can be maintained (a level similar to the mid-proliferative phase of the normal menstrual cycle). For some women monitoring can be inconvenient, because it involves frequent visits to the clinic for blood tests.

Skin gel
The most widely used form of HRT in France is a skin preparation

in the form of a gel. Oestrogel is now available in Britain. It was launched in France in 1975 and subsequently in Belgium, Luxembourg and Switzerland. The product is a hydroalcoholic gel containing 0.06 per cent 17B-oestradiol supplied in an 80-g pressurised dispenser. Each dispenser will provide at least 64 measures of 1.25 g each. The usual starting dose is 2 measures (2.5 g) of oestrogel once daily, which will provide 1.5 g of 17B-oestradiol. If after treatment for one month effective relief of symptoms (hot flushes, night sweats, genito-urinary and sleep disturbance) is not obtained this dosage may be increased to 4 measures (5 g) daily.

The lowest effective dose should be used for maintenance therapy, and in women with an intact uterus a prostogen should be used for 12 days of each month. Oestrogel should be used daily on a continuous basis. The gel is spread, after application to the arm/shoulder or inner thigh area, and allowed to dry for five minutes before any clothing contacts the skin. The gel should not be applied to the breasts or vulval area. Concomitant usage of skin preparations which may produce interaction – for example, skin cleansers and detergents, skin products containing alcohol (astringents, sunscreens and products incorporating salicylic or lactic acid) – should be avoided. Some users have reported local side effects such as irritation and reddening of the skin at the site of application. Side effects such as nausea, headache, weight gain, bloating and breast tenderness occur in about 6.5 per cent of users.

Oestrogel will improve vasomotor and genito-urinary symptoms. It is not, as yet, licensed for the prevention of osteoporosis, nor has its protective effect against cardiovascular disease been established.

Vaginal creams, pessaries and rings
These allow oestrogen to be readily supplied to, and rapidly absorbed by, the target area. However, absorption is reduced when the vaginal wall has atrophied. Substantial amounts are required initially, but as improvement occurs (for example, fewer hot flushes are experienced) applications can be reduced to two or three times weekly or even less. The ring is worn constantly and replaced every three months.

Choosing the method

How HRT is taken will depend upon personal preference and side
effects such as skin irritation from the patch, or nausea associated with
oral administration. (Side effects vary from one woman to another.)
Doctors tend to have their own preferences, too. Also, blood lipids
and clotting factors could be adversely affected, depending upon the
way the individual reacts to HRT and the dosage taken.

At present, however, the skin patch provides the best method of
achieving a circulating oestrogen level which approaches the range
found in the mid-proliferative phase of the menstrual cycle. The
patch is more expensive than oral treatment, but is more 'natural' in

Oestrogen preparations for HRT

Table 5: Individual oestrogens

Type	Generic name	Brand name
Oral		
Synthetic	ethinyloestradiol	Ethinyloestradiol
Natural	oestradiol+oestrone+oestriol	Hormonin
Natural	piperazine oestrone sulphate	Harmogen
Natural	oestriol	Ovestin
Natural	conjugated equine oestrogens	Premarin
Natural	oestradiol valerate	Progynova
Natural	oestradiol valerate	Climaval
Vaginal creams		
Synthetic	dienoestrol	Dienoestrol
Natural	oestriol	Ovestin
Natural	conjugated equine oestrogens	Premarin
Subcutaneous		
Natural	oestradiol	Oestradiol implants
Transdermal		
Natural	oestradiol	Estraderm TTS
Natural	oestradiol	Evorel
Vaginal pessary		
Natural	oestradiol	Vagifem
Skin gel		
Natural	oestradiol	Oestrogel
Vaginal ring		
Natural	oestradiol	Estring

its action because the oestrogen does not pass through the liver before being picked up by the cell surface receptors where it is needed. This may or may not be an advantage.

The comparable daily dosage levels of natural oestrogens which are considered necessary to protect against osteoporosis and coronary heart disease as well as reduce menopausal symptoms, and which most women are well able to tolerate, are natural conjugated equine oestrogen (625 micrograms orally); oestradiol valerate (1-2 mg orally); and transdermal oestradiol 17B (50 micrograms dermal patch).

Progestogens and HRT

As explained earlier in this chapter, increased thickening of the endometrium can take place when oestrogen alone (unopposed therapy) is used in HRT. Unopposed oestrogen leads to a dose- and duration-dependent increase in endometrial problems. Hyperplasia is common and can lead to cancer. In women who have not had a hysterectomy, unopposed oestrogen carries a substantial risk.

There is now convincing evidence that when a progestogen is added to oestrogen therapy the endometrium is protected from these changes. This regimen replicates what the body was doing all through the woman's fertile years: oestrogen was present in the proliferative first half of the cycle, and then the ovary added progesterone during the second half to protect the endometrium from excessive build-up and brought about a shedding (menstruation) at the correct time.

A study in the USA has shown that the occurrence of endometrial cancer in women who use opposed therapy (i.e. with a progestogen added) is significantly lower even than that found in women who are using no HRT (49 women in 100,000 as opposed to 245.5 women in 100,000).

Opposed oestrogen therapy should be used wherever oestrogen is being administered, whether orally, transdermally, as an implant or even as a vaginal cream if it is used for an extended period of time, in order to protect against endometrial hyperplasia (overgrowth of the uterine lining). The exception to this is after a hysterectomy, when oestrogen alone can be used.

The tables overleaf list the preparations available.

Progestogens available for HRT

Table 6: Individual progestogens

Type	Generic name	Brand name
Oral		
Natural	progesterone	Uterogeston (micronised)
Synthetic	medroxyprogesterone acetate	Provera
Synthetic	dydrogesterone	Duphaston
Synthetic	norethisterone	Primolut N
		Menzol
		Utovlan
Synthetic	levonorgestrel	Microval
Synthetic	norgestrel	Neogest
Injection		
Synthetic	medroxyprogesterone acetate	Depo-Provera
Pessary and suppository		
Natural	progesterone	Cyclogest

Table 7: Combined progestogen with oestrogen

Type	Generic name	Brand name
Oral	conjugated equine oestrogens+norgestrel	Prempak-C
	oestradiol valerate+ levonorgestrel	Cyclo-Progynova Nuvelle
	oestradiol+oestriol+ norethisterone	Trisequens
	oestradiol+norethisterone	Kliofem
	oestradiol valerate+ medroxyprogesterone	Tridestra
	oestradiol+ dydrogesterone	Zumenon
Transdermal	oestradiol patches+ norethisterone tablets	Estrapak-50
	oestradiol patches+ norethisterone patches	Estracombi-TTS

Progestogen dosage

The minimum daily dose required of each of the progestogens in order to produce endometrial protection over a minimum of 12–13

71

days each calendar month is as follows:

Progestogen	Dosage
natural progesterone	200-300 mg
medroxyprogesterone acetate	10 mg
dydrogesterone	10-20 mg
norethisterone	1 mg
levonorgestrel	0.15 mg
norgestrel	0.15 mg

How to take HRT

Below are two examples of an 'opposed' dosage regimen, one in which Premarin and norethisterone are taken cyclically and the other in which Estraderm skin patches and Duphaston are used cyclically:

Example 1:
    Premarin tablets 625 micrograms are taken from day 1 to day 24 inclusive in each calendar month.
    Norgestrel tablets 0.15 mg are added from day 13 to day 24 inclusive in each calendar month.

Women still having periods should start the Premarin on the first day of the period. The norgestrel is taken daily from day 13 to day 24 inclusive in the cycle.

Example 2:
    Estraderm TTS 50 micrograms is applied twice weekly from day 1 with removal of the last patch on day 24 in each calendar month (6–8 applications).
    Duphaston tablets 10 mg 1–2 daily orally from day 13 to day 24 in each calendar month.
Note: it does not matter when in the calendar month progestogen is taken, provided it is for 12 days and always at the same time in the month.

Women still having periods should apply the first patch on the first day of the period. The Duphaston is taken once or twice daily from day 13 to 24 inclusive in the cycle.

If menstrual bleeding starts prior to the last day of progestogen treatment this may indicate inadequate endometrial protection and a slightly higher progestogen dosage may therefore be required.

Some doctors prefer to prescribe calendar packs for 'opposed' regimens, but these are highly inflexible: they do not allow the dosage levels to be changed, at an early point, to suit the individual. Such tailoring of HRT is desirable because sometimes women show abnormal blood lipid changes and experience PMS-type symptoms in reaction to certain oestrogen and progestogen combinations. The PMS-type symptoms are experienced by 30-40 per cent of women on the opposed dosage regimen, at the point in the cycle when the progestogen is added to the oestrogen.

Within the last few years a more modern **alternative** approach to the above HRT regimens has been introduced. The oestrogen is taken on a continuous basis, producing a steadier blood level. The progestogen is taken for the usual 12 days.

Alternative regimen 1:
Instructions for Premarin and norgestrel are:
> Premarin: a woman who is still having regular periods should start the Premarin on the first day of the period, and take it daily on a continuous basis. A woman who has not had a period for over two months may start the Premarin at any time.
> Norgestrel (progestogen): a woman who is still having regular periods should start taking the progestogen (1 tablet daily) on day 17 of the cycle and continue until day 28. A woman who has not had a period for over two months should start taking the progestogen on the first calendar day of each month and continue until day 12.

Alternative regimen 2:
Instructions for Estraderm and Duphaston are:
> Estraderm: a woman who is still having regular periods should apply the patch on the first day of her period and change it twice-weekly on a continuous basis. A woman who has not had a period for over two months may start using it at any time.

Duphaston (progestogen): same regimen as norgestrel above, but taking 1-2 Duphaston tablets (10 mg) orally.

Nuvelle (revised form of Cyclo-Progynova) uses oestradiol valerate combined with levonorgestrel as the progestogen. One tablet is taken each day on a 28-day cycle. Menstrual bleeding takes place, usually between day 26 of one cycle and day 6 of the next. Some 'spotting' between true bleeds has been reported.

For women who do not wish to put up with the continuation of a monthly bleed after the menopause, there is a further method by which continuous combined oestrogen and progestogen therapy can be used. This opposed regimen protects the endometrium from hyperplasia, there is no bleed, and cyclic PMS-type symptoms are also often reduced. For the first few months of therapy 'tailoring' has to take place while the ideal oestrogen/progestogen combination is found.

This continuous combined oestrogen and progestogen regimen is being further developed. See 'HRT and monthly bleeds', page 78.

Two new combinations of oestrogens and progestogens in development can be taken on a continuous basis, thus eliminating unwanted monthly bleeds and at the same time giving adequate protection from osteoporosis and cardiovascular disease: conjugated equine oestrogen combined with medrogestone; and oestradiol valerate combined with cyproterone.

Distressing menopausal symptoms such as hot flushes and night sweating can be controlled using Depo-Provera (long-acting progestogen) 150 mg injected deep into the buttock muscle. This lasts up to three months. It is unlikely to remedy vaginal dryness, and what positive effect Provera may have as regards osteoporosis is in doubt: a 1991 report from New Zealand indicates that Provera used over an extended period of time (five to ten years) may have an adverse effect on bone density and, therefore, encourage the development of osteoporosis to some degree.

Possible side effects of progestogens used in HRT

Progestogens used in HRT are related structurally to either progesterone or testosterone.

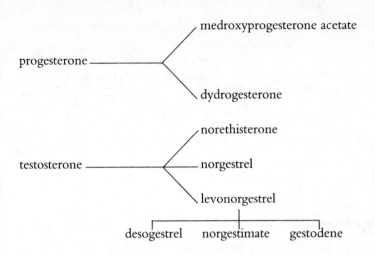

A new generation of progestogens (desogestrel, norgestimate, gestodene) derived from levonorgestrel gives rise to considerably fewer male (androgenic) characteristics and is therefore now being used in the combined oral contraceptive pill (for example, in Marvelon and Mercilon) as well as being studied for possible future use in opposed HRT.

Natural oestrogens, especially those administered non-orally, have little effect on triglyceride levels. Progestogens, especially those of high androgenic properties (norethisterone, norgestrel and levonorgestrel), tend to lower triglycerides. Depending on the type and dosage, oestrogen can lower the harmful LDL cholesterol and raise the protective HDL and HDL_2 cholesterol, but progestogens (depending on type and dosage) can work in the opposite way, thus cancelling out the benefits certain oestrogens have on lipids. Some progestogens (norethisterone, norgestrel and levonorgestrel) can cause more PMS-type symptoms than others when used in opposed HRT, including bloating, increased breast tenderness and mood swings. Dydrogesterone and medroxyprogesterone are less likely to do so.

Successful management of HRT

Finding the right combination of oestrogen and progestogen is the key to using HRT successfully. Careful management takes time and patience on the part of both patient and doctor in order to achieve the required balance of hormones which will not have adverse effects on blood lipids, blood coagulability and mood.

The introduction of the third-generation progestogens – gestodene, norgestimate and desogestrel – should make this task easier. They can reduce the negative effects that some of the progestogens in current use trigger when they are combined with oestrogens. This is in part due to the method of oestrogen administration, which in turn influences their dosage. The oral method requires higher dosages to be effective because the oestrogen has first to pass through the liver.

The benefits of HRT

- Oestrogen replacement therapy relieves menopausal vasomotor symptoms, such as hot flushes and night sweats, caused by fluctuations in oestrogen levels, and those of oestrogen lack – for example, vaginal dryness, painful intercourse and urinary frequency due to reduced muscle tone of the bladder and irritation of the lining of the bladder and urethra. The alleviation of these physical symptoms may well improve mental well-being, helping the user to avoid the anxiety and depression some women experience during the menopause and to maintain libido.
- There is evidence that HRT slows, or prevents, menopausal and post-menopausal bone loss; the reduction in the rate of bone fracture in the elderly is not yet fully known, nor is it known how long the effect lasts.
- Oestrogen in HRT protects against post-menopausal heart disease, as long as the type and strength of the progestogen used does not negate the oestrogen benefits.
- There is evidence that oestrogen replacement therapy may extend post-menopausal life expectancy and the quality of life in those years.

Reasons for not taking HRT

Absolute contraindications to HRT are few, once it has been established that there is no undiagnosed vaginal bleeding and that the patient is not pregnant. As to existing breast or endometrial cancer, there is no conclusive evidence that oestrogens produce worsening of the conditions. HRT can greatly improve the quality of life of cancer sufferers, whose life expectancy may not be very great and whose menopausal symptoms may be excessive.

Relative contraindications require careful evaluation before HRT is used, but in many circumstances therapy is both possible and safe. Specific disorders include the following:

diabetes may require re-stabilisation;

benign breast disease would require careful monitoring, but the use of HRT need not be ruled out;

otosclerosis, an unusual and possibly hereditary condition which produces hardening and fixation of the small bones in the middle ear, may be made worse with HRT according to some reports;

gall bladder disease can be adversely affected by oestrogen due to changes in bile composition and the greater risk of gall stones;

endometriosis may become worse as a result of the reactivation of the displaced endometrial tissues which oestrogen will bring about;

fibroids, which are oestrogen-dependent, may increase in size but can be monitored by pelvic examination and ultrasonography.

Varicose veins do not rule out HRT provided that they are not acutely inflamed (phlebitis). **Previous endometrial hyperplasia** should not conclusively preclude HRT provided that adequate progestogen is used (opposed therapy) and there is no previous history of endometrial carcinoma. **Liver disease** may rule out HRT, depending upon the cause and severity of the condition. However, if the uterus has been removed and the oestrogen (only) is not given by mouth – therefore bypasses the liver – HRT may be possible with careful monitoring.

There appears to be no contraindication for the use of oestrogen in patients with **hypertension** which is being controlled, or where there is a previous history of **deep-vein thrombosis**, provided that it occurred as a side effect to some other medical condition unrelated to blood disease or hormone abnormalities, or previous contraceptive usage. However, non-oral oestrogens are recommended in both cases, so that the liver is bypassed and fewer metabolic changes are incurred. The administration of HRT in such instances does none the less require very careful consideration on an individual basis, and continuous close medical monitoring. Recent deep-vein thrombosis or lung embolus would both normally preclude HRT. The extent and severity of the condition needs careful consideration and a final decision should be made according to the severity of the menopausal symptoms.

Finally, **smoking** is not a contraindication for taking HRT, but smokers are at increased risk of developing heart and circulation problems, as well as throat and lung cancer. Also, smoking accelerates the destruction of oestrogen, therefore HRT is less effective in heavy smokers. It is very important for the patient to stop smoking as the hormone changes which occur around the menopause increase the risk of many diseases.

Table 8: Contraindications to HRT

Absolute	endometrial cancer ⎫ usually but not always
	breast cancer ⎭
	pregnancy
	undiagnosed vaginal bleeding
	undiagnosed lump in breast
	present severe thromboembolism,
	e g. pulmonary embolus following hip
	replacement operation
Relative:	diabetes
	varicose veins
	benign breast disease
	previous endometrial hyperplasia
	liver disease
	gall bladder disease
	fibroids
	endometriosis
	previous or present deep-vein
	thrombosis
	hypertension
	otosclerosis

HRT and monthly bleeds

All women using HRT (except those who have had a hysterectomy) need to take a progestogen to oppose the effect of oestrogen, thus preventing any risk of excessive endometrial thickening and possible cancer. The progestogen produces monthly bleeding, however, which most would prefer to avoid.

To overcome the nuisance of monthly bleeds, new combinations of oestrogens and progestogens are being formulated. The two hormones are taken together on a continuous combined daily basis, thus protecting the endometrium from hyperplasia and reducing cyclical PMS-type symptoms.

Examples of continuous combined HRT in current use are:

(a) Premarin 0.625 mg together with Provera 2.5 mg each day.

(b) Premarin 0.625 mg together with Duphaston 10 mg each day.

(see tables 5 and 6 for generic names)

Still being sought is the ideal combination, which will prevent endometrial hyperplasia, cause no annoying 'spotting', have no adverse effect on blood lipids and cause no PMS-type symptoms but *will* protect against osteoporosis and reduce the incidence of coronary heart disease.

New oral HRT preparations

Livial (tibolone or ORG OD14), a new preparation for post-menopausal women, is the first single substance to combine the favourable effects of the three classic sex hormones (oestrogen, progesterone and testosterone). It is taken continuously and is claimed not to cause spotting, although some women using it have found this is not so. The use of a progestogen for three cycles of 12 days is recommended to diminish the endometrium before starting Livial, which is why this medication should not be used until a year after the last menstrual period.

Livial does not stimulate the endometrium, therefore regular withdrawal bleeding is avoided. It prevents ovulation, reduces the incidence of vaginal and urinary infection by improving the skin quality of those areas, as well as rendering intercourse less painful. It leaves unchanged, or improves, cholesterol and blood lipids, has no adverse affect on blood clotting factors, and reduces loss of bone density. Livial's effect on the cardiovascular system has not yet been adequately researched. The dosage is one 2.5 mg tablet daily. Symptoms are generally alleviated within a few weeks, although optimum results are only obtained after three months of continuous therapy. The incidence of reported side effects, such as spotting, is low.

The even newer **Kliofem** is the first combined hormone replacement tablet to eliminate the monthly bleed, each pill containing 2 mg of 17B-oestradiol (E_2) and 1 mg norethisterone acetate (NETA). It is licensed both for the relief of vasomotor and genito-urinary symptoms and for long-term prevention of osteoporosis.

Side effects are light irregular bleeding or spotting which may occur during the first few months of treatment. Persistent bleeding or irregular bleeding which may occur after absence of any bleeding requires investigation. Breast tenderness, nausea, headache and weight gain have also been reported. Sufferers of lactose intolerance should be aware that the tablets contain lactose as a base. PMS symptoms are noticed less frequently because the oestrogen and progestogen in Kliofem are given continuously rather than on a cyclical basis. Cardiac protection, however, has so far not been established neither has the desired increase of the protective HDL cholesterol.

The usual reasons for not taking HRT should be followed before therapy is started. A full physical to include blood pressure, breasts and pelvic examination (internal) is advisable. Kliofem is only suitable for women who have had no menstrual bleeding for at least a year.

Tridestra is the newest combined oral HRT: 2 mg of oestradiol valerate are taken daily for ten weeks. For the next two weeks daily medroxyprogesterone 20 mg is added. Bleeding occurs every 13 weeks only when no medication is taken.

PMS symptoms are reduced to four times yearly as are unwanted and annoying withdrawal bleeds. Protection against cardiovascular disease and osteoporosis is provided and menopausal symptoms are controlled.

HRT by nasal spray

Delivery of sex hormones by atomiser is being perfected. Accurate dosage of, and the vehicle used for, the hormones is crucial. Clinical trials are under way in London.

New progestogens

Friendlier, third-generation progestogens which reduce unwanted lipid side effects are currently being developed. These progestogens, such as desogestrel, norgestimate and gestodene, are being combined with oestradiol in different dosage combinations in order to give protection of the endometrium with no adverse cardiovascular effect or monthly bleeding.

Ways of giving continuous progestogen are currently being researched. An intra-uterine device (IUD) containing the progestogen levonorgestrel is available under the name of Progestoset, and an IUD with natural progesterone is produced by ALZA Laboratories. The advantage of these is that the protective influence of the progestogen/progesterone is given immediately to the uterus without having to pass through the liver first. The major disadvantage is troublesome spotting. Refinement of this method of delivering progestogen continues. It should be noted that IUDs are *not* the same as IUCDs (intra-uterine *contraceptive* devices).

New oestrogens

Oestrogens in present use are being perfected. The transdermal patch is being improved and the subcutaneous implant is being fine-tuned to lessen the high and low swings found in oestradiol blood levels with the present implant technique.

A new transdermal oestrogen in the form of a skin gel, Oestrogel, is now available (see page 68), and a nasal spray is being developed (see above).

HRT and aspirin

The relationship between HRT and blood coagulation is under constant review. Antithrombin III levels can be used to monitor increased risk of blood clots before and during HRT usage at the time of the menopause.

Fibrinogen levels rise in the blood after the menopause. Positive association has been made between a raised fibrinogen level and an increased risk of developing cardiovascular disease at the menopause and beyond. Use of fibrinogen levels to predict cardiovascular risk, however, is not practicable because of the inconsistent effects which HRT has on fibrinogen, as well as the lack of 'standardisation' existing in the laboratories able to perform the evaluation.

Recent research suggests that a 75 mg aspirin tablet taken daily while undergoing HRT may be beneficial in reducing arterial hazards. This research also links two other factors, prostacyclin and thromboxane, in the clotting process. Both are derivatives of Omega-3 fatty acids, which are found in fish oils.

Aspirin is also associated with alteration of prostaglandin formation and both are associated with cardiovascular disease. Prostaglandins in addition are involved with bone resorption. Consequently, aspirin and HRT are the focus of continuing investigation.

CHAPTER 6

CANCER RISK AND THE OESTROGENS USED IN HRT

THE relationship between oestrogen and cancer risk in the breast, endometrium, cervix and ovaries is still under active investigation.

Hormone replacement therapy (HRT) is becoming more widely prescribed, and its beneficial effects are generally agreed upon, but the possibility of adverse effects on breast tissue causes considerable concern because oestrogen plays a central role in events and changes which are also linked to breast cancer.

Breast cancer

Facts and figures (Great Britain)
- Great Britain has the highest incidence of and death rate from breast cancer in the world, Denmark the second highest
- it is the commonest malignancy in women, comprising 18 per cent of all female cancers and affecting 1 woman in 12
- in women aged 35-54, breast cancer is the commonest single cause of death
- two-thirds of breast cancer cases are diagnosed in women over the age of 50
- the incidence of breast cancer increases with age, doubling roughly every decade until the menopause, when the rate of increase reduces
- the occurrence of breast cancer in women aged 70 is approximately 10 times higher than in women aged 40

Risk factors for breast cancer

The following are currently the known and probable risk factors:
- age: as age increases, so does breast cancer risk
- reproductive hormone factors: early menarche, late menopause, no pregnancies, and late-age pregnancy are all factors which produce increased risk of breast cancer due to the increased length of time over which the breast is subjected to the influence of oestrogen and progesterone as well as other hormones produced by the ovary[1, 2]
- risk of breast cancer doubles if a woman has a close relative (mother, daughter, sister) who developed the disease before the age of 50. The risk further increases by 4–6 times if two close relatives develop the disease
- breast pain of any type is an unusual symptom of breast cancer, and only 7 per cent of women with breast cancer have breast pain as their only complaint[3]
- benign breast disease carries a slight risk depending upon the degree of breast change. For example, a slight thickening of breast tissue and simple fibroadenomas (lumpiness) produce no risk; cystic disease and complex fibroadenomas (lumpiness with other changes) show a slight risk of 1.5–2 times; breast lumps that on biopsy show abnormal cell changes (atypical hyperplasia) carry a risk of 4–5 times. However, women with both atypical hyperplasia and a close relative with known breast cancer have an absolute risk of 20–30 per cent of developing breast cancer within the next 15–20 years[3]
- weight: obesity is linked to a reduced incidence of breast cancer in pre-menopausal women, but to an increase in incidence after the menopause
- neither alcohol nor smoking appear to be implicated among the causes of breast cancer. However, women who smoke tend to have an earlier menopause (which will reduce breast cancer risk, but increase the risk of both coronary heart disease and osteoporosis)
- diet, and in particular dietary fat, does not appear to be linked to breast cancer
- radiation exposure increases the risk of breast cancer both in teenage girls and in later life, but mammographic screening is

linked to a reduction in death from cancer in women over 50
- environmental factors influence breast cancer risk: studies show that women who have moved from Japan (where death from breast cancer is the lowest in the world) to Hawaii assume the cancer rate in the host country within one or two generations[5]
- the use of oral contraceptives for four years or more by women in their early twenties or younger and before a first pregnancy increases the risk of pre-menopausal breast cancer. There is no increased risk to women who have used oral contraceptives in their late twenties and beyond for controlling pregnancy.

Women at high risk of breast cancer

In the West, up to 10 per cent of women who develop breast cancer have an abnormality in their genes (the basic unit of heredity, composed of DNA) which predisposes them to certain cancers. The presence of an abnormality in a family's genes may be suspected if:
- several cases of breast cancer exist in a family
- early onset of breast cancer in relatives occurs
- more than one type of cancer exists in family members: for example, cancer in both breasts, ovary, colon or (in males) prostate cancer. Families which do have a cancer gene frequently have members with both breast and ovarian cancer.[4]

To assess risk medical histories and hospital records are reviewed so that a family pedigree can be produced. So far two breast cancer genes, BRCA1 and BRCA2, have been isolated.

Identifying women with gene abnormalities

As more breast cancer genes are identified it will become easier to single out family members who are at risk and who carry an abnormality. If a family history and pedigree indicate susceptibility to cancer, further evaluation of risk can take place through genetic linkage analysis.

For this procedure, blood or tissue is taken from affected members of a family and markers are identified on a particular gene. Other family members at risk can then be tested for the gene abnormalities (markers) and the probability of that family member carrying the abnormal gene is confirmed.

Carriers of an abnormal breast cancer gene, which linkage analysis will help to identify, have an 80-85 per cent chance of developing the disease. Familial breast cancer is thought to have a low incidence, the BRCA1 gene abnormality being responsible for only 2 per cent of all breast cancer.

HRT and breast cancer risk

Numerous studies, 30 in fact, have been undertaken since 1980, and between 1988 and 1993 six in-depth reviews called meta-analyses.[10-15] Most of these looked at oestrogen preparations alone in relation to breast cancer risk as combined oestrogen/progestogen regimes had been used for only a relatively short period of time.

The difference in conclusions drawn from the studies and analyses may partly be due to the route by which the oestrogen is administered, for example, oral or transdermal, whether a progestogen was added and if so what type. Oestrogens taken by mouth after being absorbed pass first to the liver and cause two chemicals in the blood to be altered, sex hormone binding globulin (SHBG) is raised, and insulin-like growth factor (IGF-1) is reduced. Both are thought to provide protection to the breast against cancer, SHBG reducing the amount of oestrogen in the blood and IGF-1 through reduced stimulation of breast cancer cells. By contrast oestrogen taken by skin patch or implant has little effect on raising the protective level of SHBG and no protective lowering effect on IGF-1. Progestogens derived from testosterone (norethisterone, norgestrel and levonorgestrel) counter the beneficial rise in SHBG caused by oral oestrogens, but two progestogens — medroxyprogesterone (Provera) and dydrogesterone (Duphaston) — do not have this unfavourable effect upon SHBG.[7, 8, 9]

Enough evidence is now available for the conclusion to be drawn that HRT usage of less than ten years carries little significant risk of breast cancer. HRT usage beyond ten years may carry an extra risk of up to 30 per cent, depending on how long it is taken. This negative effect, however, is less than the risk to a woman of developing breast cancer if there was a natural *delay* of onset of the menopause.[18]

Little information is yet available on *extended* use of combined oestrogen/progestogen HRT but it seems prudent for the friendlier progestogens to be used combined with oral natural oestrogens.

The risk in using HRT long-term should be carefully weighed against the known benefits, which include:

- the potential for reducing cardiovascular death by up to 40 per cent
- protection against osteoporosis
- maintenance of satisfactory genito-urinary function
- assistance in preserving memory and ability to concentrate, as well as everyday quality of life.

Prevention of breast cancer

Women at high risk of developing breast cancer (see page 85) may also be at risk of developing other cancers and need a cautious approach to medical treatment. In addition early mammographic screening and the triphenylethylene compound tamoxifen can assist.

Mammographic screening should start at an age 5-10 years less than the youngest relative who has developed the disease. Both ultrasonography and magnetic resonance imaging associated with computer analysis are being reviewed for use in the younger woman.

Tamoxifen is being studied for long-term use for women at high risk. This 'failed contraceptive' was discarded by its manufacturer in the 1960s and then re-introduced a decade later as a means of treating cancer. Tamoxifen prevents cancer cells taking up oestrogen at the receptor level, and produces a substance called transforming growth factor B, which has the ability to reduce the growth of cancer cells. It also has the beneficial effect of reducing cholesterol and increasing bone density.

Early results of a ten-year trial in Edinburgh involving 1,600 women who had previously been treated for primary breast cancer show a 10 per cent reduction in breast cancer deaths in those taking tamoxifen, as well as a significant reduction in heart disease. Trials are now taking place to ascertain the safety of tamoxifen in long-term usage for prevention of breast cancer in women. Another trial involving a 'tamoxifen look-alike' preparation called Toremifene is taking place at the Royal Marsden Hospital, London.[19, 20, 21]

For the population at large there is currently no specific measure known to *prevent* breast cancer. Mammography is a diagnostic procedure, not a preventive one. Regular self-examination of the breasts, however, is sensible because if performed correctly it will alert women to changes in their breasts at an early stage.

Once its safety for long-term use is established, tamoxifen may be used as a preventer for breast cancer by women in their fertile years, perhaps in conjunction with an oral contraceptive. The progestogen in this contraceptive may be gestodene, the role of which in protecting against breast cancer is now being studied. It has been suggested that tamoxifen may cause some endometrial stimulation with long-term usage: gestodene's protective action upon the endometrium would allay that concern.

Antioxidants such as vitamin C, E and B-carotene (vitamin A) along with selenium have the ability to neutralise certain 'lone molecules' (free radicals) in the body which are produced from chemical reactions and can cause damage to both the endothelial lining of arteries and breast tissue.[22, 23] Research into the beneficial effects of antioxidants continues.

Retinoids, of which about 1,500 different forms are known, are chemical substances that affect the growth of certain body cells. Experiments suggest they may have a place in preventing breast cancer. Among them is 4-HPR retinamide which concentrates in breast tissue and produces transforming growth factor B, which has been shown to reduce cell growth in breast tissue.[24]

Breast cancer: slow progress towards an answer

Screening, as currently recommended, is able to reduce death from breast cancer, but not the incidence of the disease; however, screening is confined in the general population to the age group 50-64 under present NHS guidelines and, regrettably, improvements in screening techniques, surgical procedures and after-care have increased survival chances only marginally. Greater understanding of the factors which cause breast disease and the role of oestrogen and progestogens in HRT is needed. Only then can the prevention of breast cancer become a reality.

The Macmillan Fund has produced a directory for women wanting guidelines for breast cancer management. This lists cancer centres of excellence and treatment experts. Patients may consult it through their GP or by telephoning the National Health Information Service (see address section).

Endometrial cancer

In the 1960s and 1970s unopposed high doses of mainly conjugated oestrogen were used to treat menopausal symptoms in the USA. In the mid-1970s the first studies were published which linked endometrial hyperplasia and increased risk of endometrial cancer to cyclical oestrogen use. In the late 1970s it became clear that adding a progestogen to the cyclical oestrogen therapy could prevent hyperplasia of the endometrium.

Studies published in 1986[36] and 1989[37] confirm the protective effect given by the addition of a progestogen. The incidence of hyperplasia can be reduced to zero if a progestogen is added for 12-13 days of each cycle. Without added progestogens there is a duration-dependent increased risk of developing endometrial cancer which may be as high as 10-fold after 10-15 years, as indicated in two studies published in 1982[38] and 1980.[39]

A similar protective effect may be obtained with the use of a progestogen intra-uterine device which remains in place for the whole cycle and exerts its protection continuously and directly upon the endometrium, thus reducing unwanted side effects to blood fats and mood.[29]

(See 'New progestogens', Chapter 5, and 'Progestogen-releasing IUD', Chapter 8.)

Ovarian cancer

Cancer of the ovary is more common than endometrial cancer, with an incidence of 177 cases annually per million, and accounts for 6 per cent of all cancer deaths. Some 5-10 per cent of all ovarian cancer may be hereditary, and the condition is most common in white Caucasian women of higher socio-economic groups.

Ovarian cancer increases with age, and 80 per cent of all ovarian cancer is found in women over 50.

There is also a link between ovarian and breast cancer. A women with the latter has twice the normal risk of developing the former.

Studies published in 1989[40] and 1988[41] suggest that HRT appears to have no adverse effect on the ovaries. However, further studies are required before this conclusion can be confirmed.

Studies are under way, in the UK and elsewhere in Europe, to determine whether screening for ovarian cancer is both cost-effective and accurate. Two screening procedures, in combination, may be effective: evaluation of serum CA125, and colour Doppler imaging ultrasonography using a vaginal probe.

Ultimately an abnormal gene may be located, which would enable those at high risk in the population to be identified.[32]

Cervical cancer

The peak occurrence of both cervical dysplasia and cervical cancer is before the menopause.

Studies published in 1987[42] and 1989[43] found no evidence of an increase in cervical cancer with HRT. It is thought that HRT can be used safely both in women who have never been treated for cervical dysplasia and those who have.

CHAPTER **7**

Non-hormonal management of the menopause

HORMONE therapy is not the only option for managing the menopause; there are several hormone-free preparations which may be of benefit. They are, however, of limited assistance because none is able to compensate for the absence of oestrogen in the body.

Clonidine

This *may* reduce the frequency and severity of hot flushes. It will not correct or relieve other menopausal symptoms caused by lowered hormone levels. Caution has to be observed if cardiovascular or cerebrovascular disease or blood pressure problems are present. The dosage is 1 tablet of 50 micrograms twice daily. This dosage can be taken for three to six months before a break. However, clonidine is being used less and less as new studies indicate its effectiveness is low.

Anti-depressants and tranquillisers

The use of anti-depressants and tranquillisers requires extreme caution by both doctor and patient, because use can lead to abuse and dependency. Constant supervision is essential. These medications are by no means the only answer to menopause-related problems such as depression and stress, as will be seen. In fact, depression is not an automatic or typical symptom of the menopause, though some depressed women may become more so at this time.

Certainly the menopause can be a time of increased strain and stress and, on occasion, anxiety and depressed mood. A sympathetic family doctor can be of great assistance. Counselling and a reappraisal of ideas and ambitions may be more helpful in the long term than tranquillisers and anti-depressants (see page 114).

Vitamin B6 (pyridoxine)

An increase of PMS-type symptoms in the peri-menopause may be noticed as hormone swings become more frequent, whether or not a hysterectomy has been undergone. The cyclical use of progestogens with oestrogen in HRT may worsen PMS. The swings of mood, breast discomfort and aching muscles are caused by changes in the level of brain chemical messengers which are influenced by the oestrogen/progesterone balance. Some women say they have found vitamin B6, which can be bought from most chemists and health-food shops, to be of help in this respect, though a placebo response has been thought to be quite likely.

The dosage is variable, but 25-50 mg daily is considered safe; alternatively, it may be taken only during the last two weeks of the cycle (i.e. the two weeks preceding a period). Side effects have been reported with a daily dosage of over 100 mg, but these effects are more likely to occur when the vitamin has been taken for over six months. They may take the form of sensitivity of the skin to touch, weakness of muscle groups, or skin rashes.

Gamma linolenic acid (GLA)

GLA has been found by some women to be helpful in controlling PMS symptoms. GLA is a breakdown product of cis-linoleic acid (cis-LA), an essential fatty acid of vegetable origin found particularly in sunflower, safflower and corn oils. GLA is converted in the body to prostaglandins, which are able to alter body chemistry via their widespread influence upon areas such as the heart, blood vessels, intestines and arteries. Prostaglandins maintain a delicate balance with each other as well as affecting hormone relationships.

PMS is thought to be caused by hormone imbalance. It is possible, therefore, that the benefit some women perceive from taking GLA is caused by a reduction of hormone and prostaglandin imbalance as a result of GLA increasing the manufacture of prostaglandins of the E_1 series.

The dosage of GLA is variable: each woman must discover her

own benefit level. An average dosage is a 500 mg capsule taken with food (to avoid nausea) between one and three times daily for two weeks before menstruation. Efamol (brand name) contains the seed oil of the evening primrose plant *(Oenethera biennis)* and supplies 72 per cent cis-LA and approximately 10 per cent GLA; it is only one of several brands of evening primrose oil on sale at health-food shops and chemists.

Aci-Jel and K-Y jelly

Lack of oestrogen causes changes to the vagina; the walls become thinner, dryer and less acidic. This increase of alkalinity allows infections to occur. The application of acetic acid jelly (Aci-Jel) twice weekly, using an applicator, can be helpful. Replens, a vaginal moisturiser, may help. One application lasts for up to three days.

K-Y jelly is a safe lubricant for relieving vaginal dryness and making intercourse less painful.

Skin care

Cosmetic manufacturers offer a wide range of products, many of them seductively perfumed, lavishly packaged and carrying a high price tag, which they claim will prevent skin ageing. The truth is that no cosmetic can delay, let alone prevent, the ageing of the skin. However, oestrogen can improve its collagen content, and as its water content is increased and the blood flow to it is stimulated, natural wrinkles may become less obvious.

Dry skin, which becomes more apparent as the menopause nears, can easily be improved by using a simple non-hormonal skin moisturiser. The effectiveness of such a product may bear no relationship to its cost. A few years ago, the Australian Consumers Association (ACA) published formulations for skin moisturisers (see table below). These can be made up in bulk, at home, and are as effective as, and considerably cheaper than, many of the commercial preparations; they should be kept in a refrigerator in a tightly closed container.

Table 9: Skin moisturisers

For a light lotion
100 g sorbolene* (with 10 per cent glycerine)
500 ml hot water
(0.6 g benzoic acid if required)**
1.5-2 ml perfume essence (if required)†

For a heavy lotion/light cream
100 g sorbolene* (with 10 per cent glycerine)
300 ml hot water
(0.4 g benzoic acid if required)**
1.5-2 ml perfume essence (if required)†

For a mousse-type cream
100 g sorbolene* (with 10 per cent glycerine)
150 ml hot water
(0.25 g benzoic acid if required)**
1.5-2 ml perfume essence (if required)†

For a heavier cream
100 g sorbolene* (with 10 per cent glycerine)
100 ml hot water
(0.2 g benzoic acid if required)**
1.5-2 ml perfume essence (if required)†

*Sorbolene is a basic non-prescription skin cream which many dermatologists recommend for those who are allergic to perfume. It consists of 10 per cent propylene glycerol (a moisturiser) and 15 per cent non-ionic emulsifier. These ingredients are made up in water. Your local pharmacist should be able to prepare this for you in the consistency (lotion or cream) you wish.
**Benzoic acid may be added as a preservative, but even so you must store the lotion or cream in a refrigerator.
†Omit the perfume if you have allergies.

Reducing hot flushes

To help reduce the effects of hot flushes:
- wear several layers of light clothing – preferably high in cotton content – which can be adapted to the most comfortable temperature
- reduce intake of caffeine drinks and alcohol
- check with the doctor that none of the medication currently being taken is likely to induce flushes
- if reducing hormone therapy, do so slowly to avoid 'rebound flushes'
- take frequent lukewarm showers rather than a bath
- hot flushes are often worse (although not more frequent) at night:

place a soft cotton towel over the lower bed sheet (ideally also cotton) to absorb excessive perspiration and reduce the need for frequent changes of bed linen.

- reduce smoking, (and if possible, stop completely). It is reported that the first puff of each cigarette can trigger a hot flush
- try taking vitamin E, obtainable from a pharmacist or health food store, in a dosage of 200–400 iu (international units) each day (take the lowest dosage level which you find helpful) to help reduce excessive sweating and flushing. It may take three or four weeks before improvement is noticed
- take regular exercise, which should prove beneficial in reducing both the intensity and the frequency of hot flushes.

Herbal remedies

Many women find that some natural remedies help to relieve the hot flush symptoms of the menopause. These remedies include fenugreek, gotu kola, ginseng, sarsaparilla, liquorice root and tan kwai (also known as female ginseng). Preparations of camomile and other herbal teas may also be relaxing for women. Such herbal preparations are widely available from health food shops and some chemists.

It is important to realise that herbal remedies are just as likely as conventional drugs to cause side effects (asthmatics, for example, need to be wary of ginseng because of its histamine properties). There have been no clinical trials to substantiate the effectiveness of herbal remedies, but the placebo response may be strong enough to suggest that they may be the best choice for some women.

Lifestyle

A healthy lifestyle with sensible nutrition, weight regulation and regular exercise can pay amazing dividends during the peri-menopause and beyond. Peak bone mass in the pre-menopausal years will lessen the effects of the 35 per cent natural lifetime loss of cortical bone and the 50 per cent loss of trabecular bone which most women sustain (see Chapter 3). Knowing how to manage stress will mean more emotional strength during the menopausal years, and an ability to handle mood swings with minimal disruption when they do occur.

Exercise

Throughout life, exercise is important for the maintenance of bone mass and for a healthy heart and cardiovascular system. Looking after the heart and blood vessels pre-menopausally by taking adequate regular exercise and eating a sensible diet will provide a cushion of protection against cardiovascular problems which may increase at the menopause as oestrogen levels decline.

All forms of exercise are helpful. In the peri-menopause years muscle-strengthening exercises which concentrate on the large muscle groups (abdominals, back muscles and hamstrings) are particularly good. These are known as anaerobic (or isometric) exercises and, unlike aerobic exercise, they use little oxygen because the muscles move rapidly then stop. The Canadian 5BX programme (available from bookshops) is an example of anaerobic exercise.

For individuals with access to a gym, effective aerobic exercises might include walking on a treadmill or using an exercise bicycle. The treadmill and bicycle ergometer are ways of measuring fitness progress. The first calculation to gauge the initial level of fitness is the 'maximal oxygen intake' (VO_2 max). VO_2 max is estimated from pulse rate measurements during a stationary bicycle test. Average values range from 25 to 45 millilitres per kilogram per minute, which regular exercise can increase by up to 30 per cent. The aim should be to maintain the VO_2 max at an above-average level.

A personal programme can be devised which will allow the heart rate, during exercise, to be increased until the rate of 70-80 per cent of maximal rate can be maintained for 30 minutes, three or four times weekly. Maximal rate is calculated by subtracting the individual's age from 200. The type of aerobic exercise should be altered from time to time in order to reduce boredom and make the experience pleasurable; group activities such as square, ballroom and folk dancing are helpful and very enjoyable for some. Ideally, two sessions of muscular exercise and three or four sessions of aerobic exercise should be engaged in each week. (Aerobic exercise and heart rate are further discussed under 'Stress management', page 115.)

At the menopause it is wise to reduce any exercise which involves over-extending or overflexing the back (extension or flexion) to prevent any injury to the spine, which may have already been weakened. If osteoporosis is present exercise should be restricted to walking and swimming, the former with well-cushioned footwear.

Structured walking is very beneficial – for example, take a time frame of 30-45 minutes each day or every second day and divide it into three equal phases of 10-15 minutes. Phase one is warm-up; phase two is the aerobic or cardiovascular phase, when the heart rate should be maintained at a level of 200 minus your age (check this by taking your pulse); phase three is the cool-down phase, when you return to the starting point at a slow pace. Everyday exercise is useful, too: shopping, exercising the dog, climbing stairs rather than taking a lift, walking instead of using buses or a car for short distances, and so on.

Body mass index (BMI)

The ratio of weight to height, or body mass index, can be checked using tables (see table 10). BMI has limited accuracy and relevance,

Table 10: Body mass index

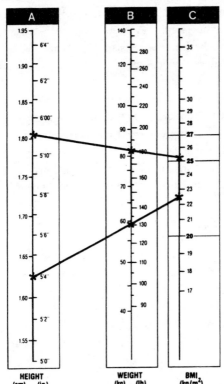

but it can give a rapid indication of health risk. The acceptable range is higher in men (20-25) than in women (20-23.5). An excess of body fat is the usual reason for a higher BMI, although the greater muscle development of those who exercise regularly may also be reflected in a higher score.

How to find your BMI

Mark an X at your height on line A, then mark an X at your weight on line B. Take a ruler and join the two Xs. To find the BMI, extend the line to line C. For example: if Michael is 5 feet 11 inches and weighs 183 lb, his BMI is about 26. If Irene is 5 feet 4 inches and weighs 132 lb, her BMI is about 23.

What the readings indicate

A BMI under 20 indicates that there may be a health risk and individuals should consult a dietician or doctor for advice. A reading between 20 and 25 indicates the healthiest range for individuals. If the BMI reading rises to between 25 and 27 it may suggest health problems for some people. A BMI of over 27 is associated with increased risk of health problems such as heart disease, high blood pressure and diabetes. It may be a good idea to seek advice from a dietician or a doctor.

Studies indicate that women with a higher-than-average BMI are protected against osteoporosis by the increased formation of oestrone (a weak form of oestrogen) from androstenedione by the fat cells (adipocytes). The reverse is seen in women suffering from anorexia nervosa or bulimia, in whom weight loss is likely to be associated with menstrual dysfunction, resulting in a tendency to osteoporosis.

Sensible nutrition

Cardiovascular disease and diet are closely linked. Various studies have recognised the association between saturated fat, blood cholesterol and coronary heart disease.

In June 1991 a consultative document called *The Health of the Nation* was presented to the British Parliament; one of its proponents – the Committee on the Medical Aspects of Food Policy (COMA) – suggests that for a healthy diet the following points should be considered:

- total dietary fat should supply less than 35 per cent of food intake energy
- saturated fats should not contribute more than 10 per cent of food intake energy
- sugary foods from non-milk sources should be reduced
- salt intake should be reduced
- starches and cereals should be increased
- alcohol intake should not exceed 14 units a week for women (see pages 111-12).

Many nutritionists recommend a diet comprising 56 per cent carbohydrate, 14 per cent protein and no more than 30 per cent total fat.

Table 11: Ideal heights and weights for women at the menopause

Height		Weight					
		small build		medium build		large build	
ft. ins.	cm	lb	kg	lb	kg	lb	kg
4 11	149.9	108	49.0	117	53.1	129	58.5
5 0	152.4	109	49.4	120	54.4	132	59.9
5 1	154.9	114	51.7	123	55.8	135	61.2
5 2	157.5	117	53.1	127	57.6	139	63.0
5 3	160.0	120	54.4	131	59.4	143	64.9
5 4	162.6	124	56.2	136	61.7	147	66.7
5 5	165.1	128	58.1	140	63.5	151	68.5
5 6	167.6	132	59.9	144	65.3	155	70.3
5 7	170.2	136	61.7	148	67.1	159	72.1
5 8	172.7	141	64.0	152	68.9	164	74.4
5 9	175.3	145	65.8	156	70.8	169	76.7
5 10	177.8	149	67.6	160	72.6	175	79.4

Carbohydrates

These take the form of simple sugars, starches and fibre. Each produces approximately 4 calories of energy per gram (as do proteins, while fats produce 9 calories of energy per gram). Sugar is not thought to be directly linked to heart disease but it does increase the chance of obesity, which in turn can magnify the risk of, diabetes, raised blood pressure and cholesterol and triglyceride levels.

Sugar

Eat as little as possible.

- Don't use sweeteners in place of sugar: they will maintain your craving for sweetness. The palate quickly adjusts to food which is less sweet (or salty).

- Add less sugar to tea, coffee, breakfast cereal and when cooking. (Best of all, do not use any.) In cooking try spices or flavourings such as cinnamon, ginger, lemon and orange instead.

- Beware of 'hidden' sugar in foods such as cakes, pastries, biscuits, 'frosted' cereals, chocolates and sweets. Remember that honey, syrups, glucose, fructose, fruit sugar, cane sugar, brown sugar, dextrose and invert sugar are all sugars. Always check food labels: the higher in the listing the ingredient appears, the higher its content in the food item.

- Beware of hidden sugar in fizzy drinks, cola, squash and some juices. Try mineral and spring water, weak tea or other infusions such as camomile and fennel. Use diluted fruit juice or low–calorie drinks.

- Cut down on jam, marmalade, lemon curd, honey, canned pie fillings and fruit in syrup. Use fresh fruits or canned fruit in natural unsweetened juice.

- Substitute complex carbohydrates (starches and fibre) for simple carbohydrates (sugars). This will help prevent constipation and reduce the risk of bowel cancer and diabetes. Blood cholesterol and triglyceride levels are often improved, too, and through reduction of blood fibrinogen (a blood protein) there is less likelihood of clotting.

Starch

The recommendation is to increase intake, by eating:

- more bread (but less 'spread'): cut thicker slices. Brown bread and heavy cereal breads, such as wholemeal, usually supply more roughage (fibre), mineral (calcium and iron) and B vitamins and also essential fatty acids (a form of polyunsaturated fat). Since 1953 all brown *and* white flours have been fortified with iron, calcium, thiamin and niacin

- more boiled and baked potatoes. Potatoes are a rich source of vitamin C, which is much reduced by the leaching of the vitamin into the cooking water if they are cut up. When boiling potatoes use a small quantity of water, add the whole potatoes with the skin intact when it is boiling, then cover tightly. Eat potatoes roasted, sautéed or as thick chips, but in moderation. Leave the peel on, for preference; it contains substantial amounts of vitamin C. Use very good hot vegetable oil, such as sunflower, corn or rapeseed for frying.

- unsugared breakfast cereals. Use grapefruit segments, sliced apple, banana or any other fruit (provided it is not overripe and therefore of a higher sugar content) to enhance the flavour
- beans, peas or lentils. They are good sources of starch and fibre.

Dietary fibre

Current advice is to include 25-30 grams per day of combined soluble and insoluble fibre in the diet. Eat a mixture of the different types of fibre-rich foods to make sure you get a variety of fibre.

Fibre, in either soluble or insoluble form, consists of complex carbohydrates which have beneficial effects on the digestive system. Many foods that are rich in starch also contain dietary fibre. **Insoluble fibre,** which provides 'roughage' or bulk, may be found in granary and wholemeal bread, the outer husks of cereals, nuts, seeds and the skins of fruit and vegetables. **Soluble fibre** is found in fruits, leafy vegetables, pulses and oats. Both forms are broken down by enzymes in the bowel and attach themselves to bile acids which contain cholesterol, preventing it from depositing itself on the walls of the arteries. Recent studies suggest that soluble fibre may reduce the blood protein fibrinogen and hence the likelihood of blood clots.

To increase fibre intake, eat:

- more bread (especially wholemeal, which contains twice as much fibre as white)
- foods made with wholewheat or wholegrains, such as wholewheat breakfast cereals (those made from corn or rice are generally very low in fibre unless it has been added); pasta (especially wholewheat pasta), brown rice (white rice is low in fibre but rich in starch); oats, including porridge, and rye bread
- more vegetables, especially peas, beans (including baked beans, but check the level for sugar content) and lentils; also leaf and root vegetables and salads
- more fruit, which provides soluble fibre in particular.

If the correct amount of fibre is being eaten, the bowels will move without effort or straining, once or twice a day, and stools will be soft and bulky.

There are negative factors to a diet containing excess fibre:

- excess gas and wind may be produced
- vitamins and minerals, especially calcium, can be poorly absorbed. The oxalic acid in spinach, and phytic acid found in *raw* bran and the tough coating of some beans (kidney, butter, broad), can reduce calcium absorption and therefore increase the risk of osteoporosis.

Protein

Proteins are complex organic compounds constructed of amino acids. There are over 20 amino acids which the body can restructure to produce others. Eight of them, however, cannot be manufactured in the adult body; these, the 'essential' amino acids, have to be ingested in the food we eat. Some foods supply complete proteins while others are incomplete, meaning that they can maintain life but lack some of the necessary amino acids required for growth, for example. When partial protein is supplemented with small amounts of complete protein, the additional amino acids are supplied. The two combine to produce balanced protein nutrition. This 'food combining' is a principle well-known to vegetarians.

The main sources of proteins are:

Complete	Incomplete
meat	peanuts
poultry	bread
fish	beans
cheese	peas
eggs	potatoes
milk	rice
	tofu (bean curd)

Adults require about 50-80 grams of protein each day. (The average Western diet contains far more protein than is necessary.) An average portion of these foods will supply the following amounts of protein per 100 grams:

meat	25 g	bread	9 g
cheese	23 g	milk	5 g
fish	20 g	beans, peas, lentils	5 g
shellfish	20 g	cereal grains	4 g
eggs	14 g	potatoes	3 g

Dietary fat

As noted in Chapter 4 on cardiovascular disease, high-density cholesterol (HDL) is protective while low-density cholesterol (LDL) is damaging. Triglycerides can influence blood clotting, and when their level is raised they may be harmful to health.

All fats contain a mixture of individual fatty acids. There are three types of fatty acids: saturated, mono-unsaturated and polyunsaturated. If the proportions of these fatty acids are unfavourable, with too much saturated fat, then the blood cholesterol tends to rise, increasing the risk of heart disease. A diet high in fat can lead to obesity, with an associated risk of high blood pressure, strokes, diabetes, gall bladder disease, arthritis and coronary heart disease, to mention just a few.

Fat in the diet may be visible, as in margarine, butter and the so-called low-fat spreads (these are still high-calorie foods), cream on milk and fat on meat. Hidden fat is found in chocolates, cakes, pastries, biscuits, mayonnaise, cheese, eggs, nuts and even avocados, which are high in saturated fat.

Reducing fat intake

The recommendations are to:

- use margarine, butter and low-fat spreads sparingly
- use less cooking fat or oil, mayonnaise and sauces
- fry less often. Poaching, steaming, baking, grilling and micro-waving are better
- trim all visible fat from meat. Skim fat from casseroles, gravies, etc
- use low-fat equivalents, both natural and manufactured, in place of fatty meats; for example, lean cuts of meat, chicken breast, tofu (bean curd), cottage cheese or pulses. Substitute cottage cheese, Edam, Camembert and reduced-fat cheese for the fatty varieties; skimmed and semi-skimmed milk, low-fat yoghurt, quark or very low-fat fromage frais for double cream
- cut down on chocolates, cakes, pastries and biscuits
- remember that polyunsaturated margarine and oils and low-fat spreads may still have a high *calorie* content.

Cholesterol

Recent concern over the association of cholesterol with heart disease has been well publicised. Some cholesterol is essential and the body independently manufactures over 1000 mg each day; so lack of dietary cholesterol should not be a problem.

It is generally accepted that in the United Kingdom most adults have too high a level of blood cholesterol, resulting from the typical Western diet which is rich in saturated fats. This can cause the liver to make more cholesterol of the harmful low-density type (LDL), which is easily deposited on the walls of the arteries, clogging them and leading to disease. Unsaturated fat, particularly polyunsaturates, can actually reduce low-density cholesterol (LDL) in the blood, and promote the production of the helpful high-density cholesterol (HDL). It is now thought that no more than 300 mg of cholesterol should be consumed daily in the diet. Most people average about 400 mg a day and should be able to reduce their blood cholesterol by changing their diet; others, however, have an inherited tendency to high blood cholesterol, and in this case medical help is required. The ideal for women in the peri-menopause is a cholesterol level approaching 5.2 mmol/L (200 mg/dl) or less. A blood cholesterol test can be requested from your doctor, who may well follow it up with advice on sensible nutrition, smoking, exercise and stress management.

A single cholesterol estimate, however, is meaningless. The significant factors are the percentages of HDL and LDL cholesterol that go to make up the total.

Reducing cholesterol
The recommendations are to:
- reduce animal fat intake by cutting down on rich dairy products and meat
- use a polyunsaturated spread instead of butter. Choose a sunflower margarine which is high in the healthy Omega-6 fatty acids
- reduce intake of egg yolks to no more than 3 per week if you have a satisfactory cholesterol level; if it is moderate to high, 2 eggs or fewer
- avoid foods rich in cholesterol, such as liver, kidney, shrimps and prawns
- increase soluble fibre intake by eating more fruit, oat cereals, peas and green beans
- consume at least 3 oily fish meals each week instead of meat (see table 12)

- make sure the diet includes plenty of vitamins C, D and A: these are thought to lower the harmful effect of blood cholesterol through their natural anti-oxidant effect on chemicals called 'free radicals' (see Chapter 6)
- have your blood cholesterol checked to produce a baseline to use for comparison purposes in the future.

Scientists are becoming more aware of the beneficial effects of both groups of fatty acids, Omega-3 and Omega-6. Each group is essential for good health, and evidence is now emerging that when combined in a balanced ratio they protect against the harmful LDL cholesterol and the risk of blood clots.

Table 12: Types and amounts of fat in fish and shellfish

type of fish	grams of fat per 100 g		
	Omega-3s	saturated	total
smoked mackerel	3.3	4.1	15.5
steamed salmon	2.9	3.4	13.0
canned sardines in tomato sauce	2.9	3.3	11.6
grilled herring	2.8	2.7	13.0
boiled crab	2.0	0.7	5.2
baked kipper	1.9	2.3	11.4
canned salmon	1.8	2.1	8.2
canned pilchards in tomato sauce	1.5	1.7	5.4
steamed trout	0.9	1.1	4.5
steamed plaice	0.4	0.3	1.9
steamed cod	0.3	0.2	1.9
steamed haddock	0.3	0.2	0.8
boiled prawns	0.2	0.3	1.0
canned tuna in brine	0.2	0.3	1.0
canned crab	0.2	0.1	0.9

Calcium

Calcium in the diet is required not only for strong bones and the prevention of osteoporosis, but also for normal blood coagulation, nerve transmission processes, and both heart and muscle action.

In early childhood the body retains 150 mg of calcium from the diet each day. In adolescence, when bone growth is at its peak, 275–500 mg of calcium is deposited in bone each day. Later in adult life bone maintenance takes over from bone growth and less calcium is needed; nevertheless, an average of 180 g is required yearly.

Calcium is absorbed mainly in the duodenum and the jejunal (first) part of the small intestine, stored in bone during the day, and released for use during the night when its normal source, food, is not available. (Women experiencing the menopause lose calcium during the night; they should have a milky bedtime drink to counteract this.)

The required daily allowance of dietary calcium has been revised upwards. International consensus is that the recommended daily allowance (RDA) of calcium is:

1000 mg/day for pre-menopausal women
1200 mg/day for peri-menopausal women
1400 mg/day for post-menopausal women

However, the RDA is under review and these figures may change.

A post-menopausal woman absorbs calcium less efficiently from the intestine and reabsorbs it more poorly in the kidneys. Higher levels of dietary calcium are therefore required. For women receiving HRT the daily intake of calcium may be lowered to 1200 mg, because oestrogen improves the absorption/reabsorption process.

Calcium is absorbed only in the 'elemental form' and several surveys indicate that only a small percentage of women take in sufficient dietary calcium on a daily basis.

Research has shown that, contrary to common belief, calcium is absorbed just as well from supplements as from calcium-rich food sources such as dairy products. An adequate supply of calcium is more important than its source. There has been a national decline in calcium uptake since the consumption of dairy foods dropped as a result of concern about their fat content.

Dietary sources of calcium
Rich sources of calcium include dairy products, bread, green vegetables, hard water, dried figs and the bones of canned sardines and salmon. Skimmed milk powder can be added to puddings and milky drinks to boost calcium intake without adding fat. Listed below is the calcium content of various foods.

Table 13: Calcium content of common foods in mg

	Quantity	mg of calcium
Dairy products		
Cheese (cheddar type)	3½ oz/100 g	800
Cheese (Camembert type)	3½ oz/100 g	380
Cheese cottage	3½ oz/100 g	60
Milk semi-skimmed	1 pint/600 ml	729
Milk full-cream	1 pint/600 ml	702
Double cream	3½ oz/100 g	50
Butter	3½ oz/100 g	15
Yoghurt	3½ oz/100 g	195
Dairy ice cream	3½ oz/100 g	140
Custard (from powder)	3½ oz/100 g	140
Cheese flan	3½ oz/100 g	260
Macaroni cheese	3½ oz/100 g	180
Cereal foods		
Milk chocolate	3½ oz/100 g	220
Plain chocolate	3½ oz/100 g	38
Sponge cake	3½ oz/100 g	140
Digestive biscuits	3½ oz/100 g	110
Muesli	3½ oz/100 g	190
Rich fruit cake	3½ oz/100 g	75
Chapatis	3½ oz/100 g	66
Bread (white)	2 oz/55 g/slice	55
Bread (wholemeal)	2 oz/55 g/slice	13
White sugar	3½ oz/100 g	2
Cornflakes	3½ oz/100 g	approx 4
Fish		
Canned sardines in oil	3½ oz/100 g	550
Canned pilchards	3½ oz/100 g	300
Cod (poached)	3½ oz/100 g	29
Cod (fried in batter)	3½ oz/100 g	80
Plaice in breadcrumbs	3½ oz/100 g	67
Kipper	3½ oz/100 g	65
Haddock (smoked)	3½ oz/100 g	58
Haddock (steamed)	3½ oz/100 g	55
Prawns boiled (weighed in shells)	3½ oz/100 g	55
Canned tuna in oil	3½ oz/100 g	7
Meat		
Pork sausages (fried)	3½ oz/100 g	55
Stewed mince	3½ oz/100 g	18
Bacon rashers (grilled)	3½ oz/100 g	13
Lambs' liver (fried)	3½ oz/100 g	12
Pork chop (grilled)	3½ oz/100 g	11
Chicken	3½ oz/100 g	10
Lamb chop (grilled)	3½ oz/100 g	9
Boiled gammon	3½ oz/100 g	9
Vegetables		
Broccoli (raw)	3½ oz/100 g	100

Spring greens	3½ oz/100 g	86
Savoy cabbage (raw)	3½ oz/100 g	75
Onion (fried)	3½ oz/100 g	61
Peanuts (roasted)	3½ oz/100 g	61
Baked beans	3½ oz/100 g	45
Potatoes (boiled)	3½ oz/100 g	4
Chips	3½ oz/100 g	14
Fruit		
Figs (dried)	3½ oz/100 g	280
Orange	3½ oz/100 g	41
Grapefruit (canned)	3½ oz/100 g	9
Pear	3½ oz/100 g	6
Apple	3½ oz/100 g	3
Banana	3½ oz/100 g	4
Grapes	3½ oz/100 g	4
Tomatoes (raw)	3½ oz/100 g	13
Drinks		
White wine (medium)	1 glass	about 14
Red wine	1 glass	about 7
Cola	1 glass	about 4
Coffee	1 cup	about 2
Tea	1 cup	less than 1

Note: 100 g is *approximately* the same as 3½ oz

Calcium supplements

If a calcium supplement is thought advisable, it is sensible to choose one that requires the least number of tablets to be taken while supplying a high percentage of 'elemental calcium' at a reasonable cost. For example:

supplement	elemental calcium available	tablets to provide 1000 mg
calcium carbonate 600 mg	240 mg (40%)	4
calcium lactate 600 mg	88 mg (13%)	12
calcium gluconate 600 mg	54 mg (9%)	17

There are other preparations, both single and combined. A doctor or pharmacist will help determine which product is the most desirable and cost-effective for you.

Because calcium is absorbed in the small intestine, it is important that any supplement should dissolve quite rapidly. This can be checked by placing a tablet in white vinegar. It should dissolve within 30 minutes. Calcium carbonate is best taken with a meal, as less gas and wind may be produced this way.

Evidence was presented at the 1990 International Conference on Calcium Regulating Hormones (held in Montreal) to the effect that calcium, whether tablets or liquid, was absorbed better from the intestine when in the citrate or malate form rather than as the carbonate. In the USA calcium is available combined with citric and malic acids in tablets and as an orange juice preparation.

Factors affecting calcium absorption
As described earlier, phytic acid and dietary oxalate (such as is found in spinach and rhubarb) reduce calcium absorption. Other dietary factors can lead to a lack of calcium. These are:

Lactase enzyme deficiency Milk intolerance is not unusual. The sufferer is unable to digest milk products because of a lack of the lactase enzyme, and this results in poor calcium absorption from the bowel, abdominal pain and diarrhoea. This deficiency of lactase, and poor lactose intake, can be overcome by eating yoghurt. This fermented product contains friendly bacteria which produce the lactase enzyme, and in turn lactose is able to be absorbed along with calcium.

Low dietary fat Vitamin D is manufactured, in part, in the skin following exposure to sunlight. In its active form (D3-calcitrol) it assists in calcium absorption. Absorption of vitamin D from the bowel is dependent upon normal fat levels in the food. In the elderly this may be defective, giving rise indirectly to poor calcium absorption and the risk of worsening osteoporosis. Some nutritionists advise a supplement of 400 iu (international units) vitamin D daily. In Britain this can be obtained from one calcium and vitamin D tablet daily.

Excessive salt intake Dietary salt, in excess, is known to increase the level of the parathyroid hormone, with a resulting increased loss of sodium from the kidneys; calcium is also lost in large quantities with it. This increased loss takes place when salt intake reaches one teaspoonful (approximately 5 g) or more daily (2000 mg sodium).

Daily requirement is approximately 500 mg sodium (1.25 g salt). (A diet high in vegetables and fruit contains a lot of potassium, which may counteract the effect of sodium.) Suggestions for reducing dietary salt are:

- read food labels before purchase and try to use products with as low a salt content as possible. Remember that sodium on the label may be shown as Na, the abbreviated chemical name
- wash frozen, canned and smoked seafood well in cold water
- wash cottage cheese in a fine-mesh sieve
- do not add salt to food
- avoid convenience foods and meals from fast-food outlets, which usually have a high sodium content
- avoid monosodium glutamate (MSG), sodium sulphate, sodium chloride and sodium nitrite, which are present in many foods
- avoid baked goods containing baking powder (sodium bicarbonate).

And if taking an antacid, check the sodium content.

Table 14: High-sodium foods and alternatives

high-sodium foods	low-sodium alternatives
Bacon, ham, bologna sausage, corned beef, frankfurters and sausages	Fresh meat and poultry
Frozen fish fillets, canned or smoked fish including sardines, salmon and herring, shellfish, shrimp, prawns and crab	Fresh fish such as cod, bluefish, salmon, sole, trout, tuna (packed in water)
Cheeses	Low-sodium cheeses; cottage cheese (unsalted or washed)
Peanut butter	Low-sodium peanut butter
Salted butter	Unsalted butter
Commercial mayonnaise	Low-salt, home-made mayonnaise
Salted nuts and dried fruit	Unsalted nuts
Baked goods	Baked goods containing sodium-free baking powder (potassium bicarbonate)
Mineral water with a high sodium content	Low-salt mineral water

Excessive protein intake Increased calcium loss is seen in those who consume excessive amounts of protein. This is thought to be due to amino acid breakdown of the protein, which adversely affects the reabsorption of calcium by the kidneys.

Lifestyle and nutrition

As observed in Chapter 1, menstrual disruption can be caused by behavioural eating disorders such as bulimia and anorexia nervosa. The anovulation which results in 40 per cent of sufferers with these disorders can lead to reduced bone mass.

Being overweight can protect against osteoporosis due to increased production of oestrone (a weaker form of oestrogen) by the fat cells. However, excessive weight causes its own risks such as hypertension and diabetes. Both smoking and alcohol consumption can adversely affect nutrition generally and, therefore, menopausal health.

Smoking

Smokers are likely to be 5-10 lb (2.2-4.5 kg) lighter than non-smokers. Smoking causes the skin to age more rapidly. It also alters oestrogen production and breakdown, and can contribute to an earlier menopause. Women taking HRT will experience less benefit from these hormones if they smoke and will therefore derive less protection against osteoporosis. Stopping smoking at the menopause could significantly reduce the risk of osteoporosis.

Alcohol

Women break down alcohol in the body in a different way from men. As a result, the ratio of alcohol level to body weight is higher than in men. Women are, therefore, more susceptible to alcoholism.

Inadequate intake of calcium and vitamin D resulting from alcohol excess and poor nutrition produces bone loss. Alcohol directly prevents absorption of calcium from the bowel and reduces bone-forming osteoblast activity, which results in loss of bone mass (see Chapter 3).

Women are advised not to consume more than 14 units of alcohol in any one week and not more than two units in any single day. One unit is the equivalent of:

- half a pint of beer, cider or lager
- a quarter pint of strong ale, vintage cider or strong lager
- a single measure of sherry, port, spirits or liqueur
- a single glass of wine.

Stress

Everyone experiences stress, but some suffer from it more often and more intensely than others. In 1950 two American psychologists classified individuals into two basic behavioural groups: Type A and Type B. In challenging situations, both displayed a predictable and characteristic 'style' in dealing with stress.

Type A	Type B
hard-driving	laid-back
achievement-oriented	easy-going
very competitive	calm
time-conscious	relaxed

The peri-menopausal years are especially stressful, partly owing to greater hormone swings but also to alterations in the family structure. It is now established that stress may give rise to anxiety and depression, is associated with coronary heart disease and can detract from the individual's sense of well-being. Recognising and coping with stress early in life will make it easier to deal with the increased strains that the menopausal years can bring.

Stress has been described as 'the extension of strain'. Up to an individual's maximal tolerance level, stress improves performance and enjoyment of life by presenting challenges that have to be met. This is a healthy balance. (Too much or too little challenge can produce imbalance in the form of 'burn-out' or 'rust-out'.) Each individual has a different tolerance level, with an upper and lower point similar to those on a thermostat. Within this range there is a 'comfort zone'; outside it some distress occurs. Distress in life is caused by 'stressors', which may be internal or external.

The key to reducing excess stress is to understand your own abilities, ambitions, habits, motives and weaknesses. By identifying your own 'comfort zone' you will be able to recognise when you are moving out of it. Analysing your lifestyle will allow you to make appropriate changes to reduce stress and thereby lessen the negative impact it may have upon you during the peri–menopausal years.

Table 15: External and internal stressors

External stressors (environmental)
- job
- unhappy marriage
- other family problems
- recent bereavement
- too much to do and too little time in which to do it
- noise
- crowding
- rapid change
- financial problems

Internal stressors (personality)
- perfectionism
- oversensitivity
- anger
- guilt
- fear
- Type 'A' personality (hard-driving, achievement-oriented, very competitive, time-urgent)

How to keep within the 'comfort zone'

The following suggestions will help you to keep within your 'comfort zone'.

- Discuss any problems that worry you with someone whom you can trust. Sayings such as 'get it off your chest' and 'a problem shared is a problem halved', while clichés, offer important advice. Talking problems through with someone can significantly reduce their impact and lessen the stress they cause.
- Have a balanced lifestyle which includes time for yourself, work, family life, hobbies, sport and exercise. Ask yourself what you don't have to do.
- Know yourself well, including your ambitions, desires and the limits of your 'comfort zone'.
- Maintain good physical health with a balanced diet, adequate sleep and regular exercise.
- Set yourself achievable and worthwhile short- and long–term goals. This will give you a sense of purpose and direction.

- Adopt a positive attitude to your capabilities and believe in yourself.
- Nurture friendship and fellowship: a partner in life who is 'a good friend' is the ideal.
- Maintain and improve your sense of humour.
- Proceed with one thing at a time.
- Listen without interrupting.
- Start the day early and avoid fighting the clock.
- Relax at some point during the day.
- Attend assertiveness training classes to assist you in coping with the excessive demands of others.

Assertiveness should not be confused with being aggressive. The essence of assertiveness is being able to value yourself, and to say 'no, thank you' when unreasonable demands are placed upon you by others.

Counselling

The task of a counsellor has been described as that of giving the client an opportunity to explore, discover and clarify ways of living more resourcefully and towards greater well-being. It can provide an opportunity to express worries about the menopause and the years ahead as well as to discuss more general questions about the pattern and direction of the individual's life. It is also a good way of finding out which situations cause the most stress; a counsellor can often point out factors of which an individual may be unaware and suggest ways of mitigating the pressures they bring.

Numerous organisations, including special menopause clinics, offer counselling. Addresses are given at the end of the book.

Stress management through relaxation

Relaxation can be achieved by any of these methods.

- Focusing your attention on an object or other focal point and breathing in and out slowly and evenly.
- Muscle group relaxation: progressively tensing then relaxing groups of muscles in sequence.
- Mental imagery: concentrating on a soothing or relaxing scene.
- Standard autogenic training (SAT) (see below).

While the first three methods are self-explanatory, SAT deserves explanation. Standard autogenic training is widely used in Europe and Japan, and has come to the forefront of stress management in

North America during the last ten years. Participants are trained in six standard exercises; intrinsic to these are a feeling of warmth and heaviness in the extremities of the body, warmth in the abdomen and a feeling of coolness about the forehead. Along with slow, deep breathing and reduced heart action, long-term conditioning of the nervous system is created. The 'flight and fright' response to strain is replaced by the calmer, controlled relaxation response.

SAT has been shown to achieve significant reduction in feelings of tension and depression, proving that stress can be altered by behavioural modification.

The corticotrophin release hormone, CRH (page 35), plays an essential role in enabling the body to withstand stress, by increasing heart rate, respiratory rate and circulating blood sugar levels.

Sometimes the system malfunctions: over-activity can lead to severe depression, anorexia nervosa, panic and obsessive-compulsive disorders, all of which may be regarded as maladaptive reactions to stress. CRH is found not only in the brain, but also in body tissue. Females make more tissue CRH than males and research has shown that oestrogen 'switches on the gene' which activates the CRH. The immune system is stimulated by CRH, increasing the number of white blood cells at sites of local tissue inflammation. This is why women are more likely to develop inflammatory diseases linked to the immune system (auto-immune disease), such as rheumatoid arthritis and lupus, than men.

Stress management through exercise

Exercise is beneficial in the control and modification of stress. It improves the cardiovascular system, strengthens the heart muscle and reduces the harmful effects of low-density cholesterol (LDL) by inversely increasing the level of the protective high-density cholesterol (HDL) in the blood. Exercise also improves the oxygen supply to the brain, while increased muscle action massages certain organs and better nutrient absorption from the intestine is brought about by improved and more rapid blood supply. All these effects are beneficial in the peri-menopausal years.

A word of caution: before embarking on an exercise programme, it is advisable to undergo a medical check and physical examination to establish the health and strength of the cardiovascular system, spine, ankle and knee joints.

Exercise also plays its part in maintaining a good appearance and preventing undue weight gain. But beware! Society today is obsessed with thinness. Eating disorders such as anorexia nervosa and bulimia are quite common, and may lead to menstrual disorders and osteoporosis. Excessive exercise can cause similar changes in hormone levels and, again, the risk of osteoporosis. Moderation, therefore, is essential: enough is good, too much is harmful. A sensible approach is needed.

It is important that any exercise programme should be fun – something to look forward to. Try to set aside a certain time each day. Mornings, when you are at your freshest, are usually best but that will depend upon your lifestyle and working schedule. Always begin a programme slowly – start with 5-10 minutes each day and gradually work up to an hour. Try to vary the type of exercise.

Callisthenics may be done at any time of the day when you need a boost. They include sit-ups, knee-bends, toe-touching, arm circles, head rotations, side-bends, arm twists, knee-ups and leg lifts. This tones up muscle groups and stretches muscles and ligaments.

Aerobic activities such as jumping, dancing, kicking and skipping exercise specific muscle groups and improve general flexibility. These raise the heart rate to about 120 beats per minute. Ideally they should be done for 15-20 minutes about 3-4 times weekly. Commence by exercising for 3-4 minutes only at each session, slowly increasing until you reach your goal, which should be within 8-10 weeks.

Aerobics classes have become very popular. Typically, classes last for approximately 45-60 minutes and are held three times weekly. Ideally the session should consist of a 10-15-minute warm-up of stretching exercise, similar to callisthenics, followed by 5-10 minutes of sustained high-intensity aerobic activity – often called cardiovascular exercise, because the heart is the principal target of the exercise pattern. This should be followed by 10-15 minutes of cool-down exercises. The classes are directed by an instructor who leads the group, usually in time to music.

Aerobics class injury risk is reduced if you:
- select an instructor and organisation with a good programme and reputation. The instructor should have a certificate from, or be a member of, a recognised national organisation. Contact the Central Council of Physical Recreation (see address list)

- start slowly and gradually increase your exercise time
- choose a good pair of cushioned, supportive exercise shoes
- have adequate warm-up and cool-down periods
- have a periodic safety monitoring and pulse check during the work-out.

Other excellent forms of aerobic exercise are fast walking, swimming and bicycling. Fast walking is probably the best and safest exercise of all; it imposes only about a third of the impact stress on the knees caused by jogging, for example. However, the most likely cause of injury is pushing yourself beyond a pleasant level of tiredness. Remember to start slowly, and pace yourself.

Alternative forms of relaxation therapy

Many forms of therapy are now available and it is a matter of individual choice as to which to practise; finding the right one may take some experimentation. The important thing is to find a practitioner whom you trust and feel at ease with. In Britain, there are neither laws governing the practice of complementary medicine, nor any centralised training. Most complementary therapies, however, have their own representative bodies which provide guidelines and will supply the public with lists of therapists.

Acupuncture and acupressure

Acupuncture and acupressure are ancient forms of Chinese medicine which are now sufficiently popular in the West to be available in most cities and towns. The most important literature on acupuncture is to be found in the 34 volumes of the *Nei Ching*, which was written over a period of 1,500 years and completed about 3,000 years ago.

Chinese philosophy is based on the belief that there is a life force, called *chi*, composed of two flows of energy, *yin* and *yang* (negative and positive). These energies should flow freely, in balance with one another, through channels in the body called meridians. When a flow is blocked or unbalanced, disease results. There are 26 major meridians, each of which is associated with an organ or a body function, and the acupuncture points (of which there are about 1,000) are where these emerge at the surface of the body.

An acupuncturist will take a patient's history, feel the pulse in the wrist which relate to the internal organs and probably look at the tongue before inserting any needles. Fresh needles are unsealed for each patient and disposed of afterwards. The needles are normally inserted just under the skin and the patient feels only a slight pricking sensation; there may be some discomfort when the acupuncturist decides to place the needle deeper. Very often an immediate sense of relaxation and well-being results.

Acupressure is based on the same principle of energy flow, but the points are massaged with finger or thumb, making it possible to perform on oneself.

A list of registered acupuncturists can be obtained from the British Medical Acupuncture Association (see address list).

Alexander Technique

The Alexander Technique was developed by an Australian actor, Frederick Matthias Alexander, who suffered a recurring problem of loss of voice on stage. He discovered that the root of the problem was that tension caused him to hold his body in such a way that his breathing, and therefore his voice, was affected. He went on to explore the significance of this in relation to the whole body and subsequently began to teach his findings in 1894.

The theory upon which the technique is based is that use affects structure, which in turn affects the quality of a particular function. An Alexander teacher will look at the habits of use that predispose a pupil to neuromuscular tension, which can lead to a variety of disorders. It is often thought that the purpose of the Alexander Technique is to teach good posture, but this is not the case. However, it is true to say that posture changes as use and function change.

In an Alexander Technique lesson the teacher will gently manipulate the pupil's body and ask the pupil to stand, sit and walk around. Meanwhile, the pupil will be encouraged to develop an awareness of unnecessary tension or effort that may accompany simple movements. Having recognised bad habits, the pupil will learn to change them.

The course of lessons may extend to 30 or more while the pupil learns new techniques of movement. Initial success may be difficult to detect, although sometimes improvement is almost instantaneous. Alexander Technique teachers undergo a three-year training under the auspices of the Society of Teachers of the Alexander Technique, after which they are issued with a certificate of authority. Details can be obtained from the Society by sending a 9 x 6 inch (22 x 15 cm) s.a.e. to the address at the back of the book.

Aromatherapy

Aromatherapy is the use of essential oils to restore the body's natural rhythm. These oils are extracted or distilled from different parts of flowers, trees, herbs and fruit. They can be used in compresses, in baths and as inhalants, but probably the most pleasurable and relaxing way of receiving their benefits is to be massaged with them. Aromatherapists believe that the essential oils can affect body and mind, both through inhalation and through the skin, and it is certain that the kneading of the body that takes place during massage is in itself beneficial in that it improves the circulation of the blood and lymph fluid.

For a list of registered aromatherapists, send an s.a.e. to the International Federation of Aromatherapists, which is a representative, but not a licensing, body (see address list).

Body massage

Massage is the most familiar soft tissue technique. Muscles, tendons and ligaments are mobilised by the therapist's hands and fingers in order to induce relaxation, increase local circulation and movement and relieve pain. Massage is usually used in conjunction with essential oils (see also Aromatherapy).

Reflexology

The principle behind reflexology is that each part of the body is linked to a particular zone of the hands and feet. When the zone is stimulated by massage, the corresponding organ is affected. If pain is felt it means there is a blockage or disturbance in the life flow to the organ. Reflexology is nearly always relaxing, and it maintains health by improving circulation and lymph drainage.

Further information can be obtained from the British School of Reflexology (address at the back of the book).

Shiatsu

Shiatsu is a Japanese therapy which applies stretching and pressure throughout the body to the same meridians as are used in acupuncture. The therapist uses the fingers, thumbs, palms, elbows, knees or feet to stimulate blood and lymphatic fluid circulation, release waste products that have built up in the muscles and promote relaxation.

For a list of licensed practitioners of shiatsu, send an s.a.e. to the Shiatsu Society (address at the back of the book).

T'ai Chi

T'ai Chi uses body movements to promote health of mind and body. In physical terms, it helps to relax the whole body and to deepen breathing, to improve co-ordination, to loosen joints, increase flexibility, and – in more subtle terms – it teaches self-control and develops patience and perseverance. The movements are rhythmic cycles with a constant fluid shifting of body weight, with spiral movements of the arms. To the onlooker it appears as a gentle, contemplative slow-moving dance. Unlike yoga, there is no holding of postures and no stretching. T'ai Chi is best learnt by class attendance.

Yoga

Yoga originated in India some 3,000 years ago. It combines an improvement in physical health with that of mental well-being, the belief on which it is based being that most ailments are caused by wrong posture, wrong diet and wrong mental attitudes. The physical exercises are performed slowly and gently, and should never demand effort or cause strain. Consequently, no level of fitness is required to embark upon them. Breathing, relaxation and concentration exercises are normally also included in a yoga class.

Lists of yoga groups can be obtained from the British Wheel of Yoga (address at the back of the book).

CHAPTER 8

CONTRACEPTION AND THE MENOPAUSE – PRESENT AND FUTURE

THE MENOPAUSE is a point in time when the last period has taken place, the event being noted retrospectively.

Contraception must be both effective and safe. Ideally, during the last 10 years of fertility it should also incorporate some hormone replacement to protect against the pelvic disorders which may occur in this phase of life. Declining ovarian function with consequent episodes of anovulation (lack of ovulation) leaves the endometrium exposed to unopposed oestrogen action, which may result in endometrial hyperplasia and possible cell change. Hormone-linked contraception can prevent this, protect against osteoporosis and reduce any distressing pre-menopausal symptoms.

Older women can gain more non-contraceptive benefits from the combined oral contraceptive pill (COC) than younger women. COCs will give considerable protection from heavy irregular menstrual bleeding, fibroids, benign breast disease, and PMS, all of which may increase as the menopause approaches. COC usage in the later fertile years on the run-up to the menopause will give significant protection from ovarian and endometrial cancer while producing no extra risk for developing breast cancer.

Pregnancy after 40

Fertility starts to decline in the third decade and is 20 per cent less in the fourth decade than it was in the second.

Twenty-five per cent of pregnancies in women over the age of 40 end in a spontaneous abortion. There is also a greater risk of foetal abnormalities such as Down's syndrome (and a consequent risk to the woman which arises from a therapeutic termination of the pregnancy). Over 40 per cent of all conceptions in those over 40 are terminated for one reason or another. It is wise, therefore, for women to continue to use contraception for one year following the last menstrual period unless they are prepared to undertake a late pregnancy with its consequent risks.

Table 16: Combined oral contraceptive pills

Generic name	Brand name	Dosage		
		Oestrogen (mcg)	Progestogen (mg)	
Combined				
Ethinyl oestradiol/	Loestrin 20	20	1	norethisterone acetate
norethisterone type	Loestrin 30	30	1.5	norethisterone acetate
	Conova 30	30	2	ethynodiol diacetate
	Brevinor	35	0.5	norethisterone
	Ovysmen	35	0.5	norethisterone
	Neocon 1/35	35	1	norethisterone
	Norimin	35	1	norethisterone
Ethinyl oestradiol/	Microgynon 30	30	0.15	
levonorgestrel	Ovranette	30	0.15	
	Eugynon 30	30	0.25	
	Ovran 30	30	0.25	
	Ovran	50	0.25	
Ethinyl oestradiol/	Mercilon	20	0.15	
desogestrel	Marvelon	30	0.15	
Ethinyl oestradiol/	Femodene	30	0.075	
gestodene	Minulet	30	0.075	
Ethinyl oestradiol/	Cilest	35	0.25	
norgestimate				
Mestranol/	Norinyl-1	50	1	
norethisterone	Ortho-Novin1/50	50	1	
Biphasic and triphasic				
Ethinyl oestradiol/	BiNovum	35	0.5	(7 tabs)
norethisterone		35	1	(14 tabs)
	Synphase	35	0.5	(7 tabs)
		35	1	(9 tabs)
		35	0.5	(5 tabs)

	TriNovum	35	0.5	(7 tabs)
		35	0.75	(7 tabs)
		35	1	(7 tabs)
Ethinyl oestradiol/ levonorgestrel	Logynon 30	0.05	(6 tabs)	
		40	0.075	(5 tabs)
		30	0.125	(10 tabs)
	Trinordiol	30	0.05	(6 tabs)
		40	0.075	(5 tabs)
		30	0.125	(10 tabs)
Ethinyl oestradiol/ gestodene	Tri-Minulet	30	0.05	(6 tabs)
		40	0.07	(5 tabs)
		30	0.1	(10 tabs)
	Triadene	30	0.05	(6 tabs)
		40	0.07	(5 tabs)
		30	0.1	(10 tabs)
Progestogen only				
Norethisterone type	Micronor	–	0.35	norethisterone
	Noriday	–	0.35	norethisterone
	Femulen	–	0.5	ethynodiol diacetate
Levonorgestrel	Microval	–	0.03	
	Norgeston	–	0.03	
	Neogest	–	0.075	norgestrel

Menopausal disorders and hormonal contraception

Certain disorders are particularly common in the fourth decade and beyond, partly owing to age, partly because of hormone fluctuations. Their occurrence can be reduced with carefully supervised hormone therapy, but on occasion surgical intervention may also be required. They are: heavy bleeding, with or without pain, and irregular bleeding; premenstrual syndrome; endometriosis (a disorder in which endometrial tissue forms outside the endometrium, causing pain); uterine fibroids; sexual dysfunction; endometrial hyperplasia, possibly leading to cancer of the uterus; and ovarian cancer.

Contraceptive choices

HRT preparations are not suitable as contraceptives because their hormone dosage level is intended simply to replace the body's dwindling supply, not to encourage the hypothalamus to suppress ovulation, which requires higher dosage levels.

The newer combined oral contraceptive pills (COCs) use lower levels of oestrogen, in the form of ethinyl oestradiol, combined with a new generation of progestogens. Safer contraception in the form of these lower-dosage pills helps bridge the gap between the early peri-menopause and the menopause; for most women this means the decade from age 40 to age 50.

The USA Food and Drug Administration and Maternal Health Drug Advisory Committee recommended in 1989 that there should be no upper age limit for oral contraceptive usage by 'healthy non-smoking women'. This careful landmark decision cleared the way not only for oral contraceptives to be taken by over-40s, but also for other, non-oral hormonal methods to be used; because these are non-oral, drug passage through the liver is avoided and lower dosage levels are needed.

The combined oral contraceptive pill (COC)

Modern COCs now offer safe contraception until the menopause. Their hormone content offers protection against osteoporosis up to the menopause, when HRT therapy using lower doses of different oestrogens, and in some cases protestogens, can take over. (The relative potency of ethinyl oestradiol in any COC is 1,000 times greater than 17B-oestradiol as delivered by transdermal skin patch in HRT.)

Modern COCs (for example, Minulet, Femodene and Marvelon) usually contain 0.3 mg of ethinyl oestradiol, but an even lower level of 0.2 mg is found in Mercilon. Both Marvelon and Mercilon incorporate the lipid-friendly desogestrel as the progestogen, and Minulet and Femodene contain gestodene.

Although there is still some concern that using COCs before the age of 25 may increase the risk of breast cancer, there is no evidence of increase in the risk of breast cancer where they are used after the age of 25, or after the first pregnancy.

Smoking significantly increases the risk of blood clotting, which is why COCs are not recommended for any woman over the age of 35 who smokes.

Contraindications for taking COCs

COCs are inadvisable for women with:

(1) past or present disease influencing the circulation, such as:

  (a) thrombosis

  (b) stroke

  (c) migraine of the 'focal' or 'crescendo' type

  (d) any disease, condition or habit which makes blood clotting more likely: abnormal blood lipids, diabetes mellitus, high blood pressure, irregular heart action, heart valve disease, angina, sickle cell anaemia, leukaemia and polycythaemia, collagen diseases, long-term bed confinement, smoking, obesity; COCs should also not be taken within two weeks, before or after, of a planned surgical operation

(2) past history of cancer where the pill hormones may worsen or exacerbate the condition

(3) diseases of the liver:

  (a) previous or present hepatitis

  (b) previous jaundice of pregnancy

  (c) cirrhosis and liver tumour

  (d) porphyria

  (e) bile excretion problems

  (f) known gall bladder disease

(4) disease of the pituitary gland

(5) undiagnosed vaginal bleeding

(6) actual or possible pregnancy

(7) any serious condition in the past which worsened during pregnancy and was known to be linked to sex hormones

(8) any condition present which occurred primarily as a result of taking the pill

(9) history of past hydatidiform mole (abnormal development of pregnancy where there is no foetus, just overgrowth of the placenta).

Table 17: How to take the combined oral contraceptive pill

Starting the pill

Start the course on the first day of your period. You are safe from the first pill you take. Finish this packet after 3 weeks and begin the next packet exactly a week later. (Start each new packet on the same day of the week.) Your first pill period therefore comes after 3 weeks, not 4.

Missed or forgotten pills

If you miss the pill for more than 12 hours take the missed pill when you remember and the next pill at the usual time. Use additional precautions (e.g. a condom) for the next seven days. (If these seven days run beyond the end of your packet, start the next packet straight away – i.e. do not have a gap between packets.)

Certain medicines (e.g. antibiotics) can affect the efficacy of the pill so always tell your doctor you are on the pill when he or she is prescribing for you.

Vomiting and diarrhoea can also affect the efficacy of the pill, so additional precautions (e.g. a condom) must be used while the symptoms last and for up to 7 days after they have finished.

Advantages of COCs

- 99 per cent effective in preventing pregnancy
- regularise menstrual periods, reduce cyclical bleeding by 50 per cent and give protection from menstrual problems
- give protection against endometrial and ovarian cancer
- give some protection against osteoporosis.

Disadvantages of COCs

- increase risk of venous blood clots, stroke and cerebral blood clots
- may increase blood pressure
- may predispose the cervix to cell change with prolonged usage
- may increase breast cancer risk with early use.

The disadvantages listed above are in the main quoted from studies of the older COCs. Modern COCs carry less risk, but to what degree is not yet known. However, they may reduce the blood-clotting risk.

The Schering Drug Company, which launched the low-dosage

COC Femodene in the UK in 1987, is running the world's first clinical trial to discover whether gestodene, the progestogen in Femodene, can retard growth of breast cancer cells. The company reports that recent laboratory work both at King's College Hospital, London and at the National Cancer Institute in the USA has shown that gestodene is able to reduce breast cancer cell growth. It is possible, therefore, that the incorporation of this drug in a modern COC such as Femodene might prevent breast cancer to some degree.

Modern COCs, as confirmed in a recent study, produce no more than 1-2 lb in weight gain in women over 30 years. Nausea, depression, fluid retention and headache are also much less in evidence when the oestrogen content is less than 50 mcg and the progestogen is one of the newer friendlier forms.

COCs and the menopause

Women taking the COC pill will not know whether they have reached the menopause unless they stop taking it and switch to a barrier method (see pages 134-8). A good time to make the switch is at age 50. Vasomotor symptoms (flushes, sweats and so on) may then be noted, within less than a month from the withdrawal of the oestrogen contained in the COC. If after one to three months a blood test is taken and a high follicle-stimulating hormone level is noted, this is a strong indication that the menopause has taken place. Further ovulation is now unlikely, though not completely impossible. The decision to start HRT or not should now be taken, but contraception, using a barrier method, should in any case be continued for a further year.

If, however, when the COC is discontinued the follicle-stimulating hormone level is found to be normal or menstruation re-starts, this means that some degree of fertility is still present. Contraception should therefore be continued, by a barrier method, or using a spermicide or sponge.

The progestogen-only contraceptive pill (POP)

These are often prescribed in cases where the combined oral contraceptive pill is ruled out, but careful consideration must be given to their usage in relation to other risks. After such deliberation, they may be used where there is:

(1) a family history of disease of the circulation, such as thrombosis, including deep-vein thrombosis

(2) diabetes

(3) high blood pressure

(4) heavy cigarette-smoking (over 15 per day)

(5) age over 40

(6) long duration of COC usage before the age of 35

(7) obesity

(8) severe PMS

(9) fluid retention

(10) depression

(11) concomitant use of drugs used to treat TB and epilepsy

(12) abnormal cervical smears, present or past

(13) breast cancer (short-term use only until more data is available)

(14) simple surface varicose veins.

Special medical supervision is required if the POP is prescribed in any of the above circumstances. However, many women transfer to the POP from the COC to alleviate the COC's common side effects, such as weight gain, nausea, depression, fluid retention and headache. Preparations in common use are shown below.

Table 18: Progestogen-only contraceptive pills

Generic name	Brand name	Dosage
levonorgestrel	{ Microval Norgeston	30 mcg
norgestrel	Neogest	75 mcg
norethisterone	{ Micronor Noriday	0.35 mg
ethynodiol diacetate	Femulen	0.50 mg

POPs can be used up to the menopause and are effective in 70 per cent of users for controlling some menopausal symptoms as well as PMS. (A higher dose of progestogen is usually required to prevent hot flushes.)

The POP has a low failure rate (generally fewer than four pregnancies per 1,000 users per year), but *must* be taken conscientiously on a daily basis. Cessation of periods (amenorrhoea) is common beyond the age of 45 and so is annoying 'spotting'. Cysts on the ovaries can also occur. Those with no monthly bleeding may wonder whether they have reached the menopause; this can be determined by having a blood test to estimate the level of follicle-stimulating hormone. The follicle-stimulating hormone level is checked while the method is being continued. If the follicle-stimulating hormone level is low, the POP should be continued. If it is high and vasomotor symptoms are present, and if a further check on the follicle-stimulating hormone level three months later shows that it remains high, contraception can be discontinued, or for extra peace of mind a barrier method used.

Younger women, and those requiring extra reassurance, should continue to use a simple contraceptive method (barrier, spermicide or sponge) for one year after the last spontaneous bleed.

How the progestogen-only pill prevents pregnancy

- It alters the natural progesterone effect upon the endometrium, making it inhospitable to the ovum.
- It interferes with the normal muscular action of the Fallopian tubes and hinders the journey of the ovum from ovary to uterus.
- It adversely changes the quality and quantity of the cervical mucus.

Such alterations to normal body function hinder movement of the sperm from the vagina to the point where fertilisation of the ovum takes place.

Table 19: How to take the progestogen-only contraceptive pill

---

Starting the pill
 Start the packet on the first day of your period. You will be safe straight away. Take it every day without a break and at exactly the same time every day or within 3 hours of this time.

Missed or forgotten pills
 If you miss the pill for more than 3 hours, take the missed pill when you remember and the next pill at the usual time. Use additional precautions (e.g. a condom) for the next 48 hours.
Vomiting and diarrhoea can affect the efficacy of the pill, so additional precautions (e.g. a condom) must be used while the symptoms last and for up to 48 hours after they have finished.

Other non-oestrogen contraceptive methods

There are at present four other methods of contraception where progestogens are used. Better systems of delivery of the newer progestogens are being developed in an attempt to improve efficiency and avoid the necessity of their passage through the liver. Further advantages are that the duration of action is extended, blood levels are continuous and steady and they are more pleasant to use. Possible disadvantages are irregular bleeding patterns, amenorrhoea, and occasionally facial acne.

The four methods being used as alternatives to the progestogen-only pill are: injectables; subdermal implants; vaginal rings (not yet widely available); and progestogen-releasing intra-uterine contraceptive devices (IUCD) (also not yet widely available).

Progestogen injectables

Generic name	Brand name	Dosage
Medroxyprogesterone acetate (MPA)	Depo-Provera	150 mg intramuscularly in a watery solution every three months
Norethisterone oenanthate (NET-OEN)	{ Noristerat Norigest	200 mg in an oily solution every two months

Both drugs inhibit ovulation. Mood swings and some weight gain are possible side effects.

Depo-Provera (not approved in the USA for long-term contraceptive use) is used in the UK and other countries as a contraceptive (though comparatively rarely in the UK). It is taken once every three months, so it has the advantage of convenience and is likely to appeal to forgetful users, as well as those who dislike having to 'pop pills' on a daily basis. Spotting can be troublesome, and there is also the possibility of increased risk of osteoporosis.

Subdermal implants

In 1964 Folkman and Long pioneered research into the passage of steroids through silicone rubber. In 1967 Segal and Croxatto showed that when a progestogen is placed in silicone rubber capsules and placed beneath the skin it can be used for long-term contraception. The idea was marketed as 'silastic' capsules using levonorgestrel as the progestogen. The implant is available as Norplant; a refined method, Norplant-2, is not available in the UK at the time of writing.

The sustained release system consists of six silastic capsules which are placed subdermally, under local anaesthetic, on the inside of the non-dominant upper arm. The reason for using the non-dominant arm is that its lesser degree of muscle movement will minimise the chance of extrusions. This implant will give a high degree (98 per cent) of pregnancy protection for up to five years.

The effectiveness of Norplant-2 is the same as that of Norplant; however, two capsules in rod form, instead of six, are implanted.

Both insertion and removal require the skill of a trained professional. The capsules are placed below the skin surface in a fan-shaped fashion under local anaesthesia. Insertion usually takes 10-15 minutes and removal, again under local anaesthesia, 15-20 minutes. Fertility returns within a few weeks of Norplant removal, much faster than when Depo-Provera or oral contraception are stopped.

Both systems may give rise to bleeding irregularities along with amenorrhoea; these usually normalise with time. Other problems are unusual because of the low dosage of levonorgestrel used; however, headache, dizziness, weight change, depression and acne eruptions have all been reported. The incidence of ectopic pregnancy (where the egg is fertilised and embeds itself in the Fallopian tube) is lower than that in women using no contraception.

Before opting for such a method it is important to have adequate counselling so that the benefits, the possible side effects and the placing and removal of the delivery system are fully understood.

The future: implants, vaginal rings and IUCDs

Following the success of the levonorgestrel implant system, new directions in slow-release mechanisms are being studied. The aim is to produce 'friendlier' progestogens with more progesterone action and less androgen (masculinising) effect. Those being produced from levonorgestrel (such as gestodene) are of this type.

Implants

The pure progesterone implant
This provides effective contraception for up to five months using six pellets compressed into a single cylinder 11.8 mm in length and 3.2 mm in diameter. There is, however, a high rate of cylinder and pellet extrusion – that is to say, the cylinder/pellet is pushed out to the skin surface. Refinement is required to overcome this.

The ST-1435 implant
This derivative of 19-nor-progesterone is contained in a silastic capsule. One capsule suppresses ovulation for up to six months, while five capsules give contraceptive cover for up to 18 months. The major drawback is abnormal bleeding patterns, and a shorter duration of effectiveness than that of Norplant. A new release system is being studied.

The ketodesogestrel implant
This progestogen is the breakdown product of a third-generation progestogen (desogestrel) which is currently in use in the COC Marvelon. The silastic capsule prevents ovulation and is effective for up to two years. A side effect is menstrual irregularity. Efforts are under way in the UK, China and Sweden to perfect the system.

Capronor implant and fused pellets
These are under investigation and could be available for use in the late 1990s. Both are bio-degradable (they break down and are absorbed after a few years). Both systems are recoverable during the first 18-24 months prior to the start of the disintegration process. Capronor contains levonorgestrel while the pellets incorporate norethisterone fused with cholesterol. Again, irregular menstrual bleeding is the main side effect, but both provide highly effective contraception.

By the end of the decade improved implants which are effective for one to five years will be on the market. They may prove to be the first choice of contraception for many women in the future.

Vaginal rings

The use of silastic as a reservoir for bringing hormones into contact with the vaginal mucous membrane is being developed. This has the advantage of using natural oestrogen and progesterone under the control of the user, in other words, the user may remove the device when she wishes, which is not possible with injectable or implanted contraceptives : vaginal rings, for example, Estring, may also be used for delivering HRT in the menopause.

The World Health Organisation is currently developing a progestogen-only ring using levonorgestrel which, after insertion, is left continuously in the vagina. Another ring using both a progestogen and ethinyl oestradiol, in different sections of the device, is also being tested. It is used cyclically, being left in place for three weeks then removed for one. This may become an alternative to the low-dosage COC pill.

Progestogen-releasing IUCD (LNG IUD)

The LNG IUD Mirena, a promising Swedish-Finnish method of contraception, has recently gained regulatory approval in the UK. A silastic capsule containing a progestogen (levonorgestrel) is incorporated into the stem of an intra-uterine device. Its slow-release delivery lasts up to five years. There is a marked reduction in menstrual blood loss, although spotting may occur for the first three months after insertion. Pelvic infection is minimal and neither blood pressure nor body weight is affected. Published studies covering over 10,000 woman-years indicate a pregnancy rate of under 0.2 per 100 women.

Because the LNG IUD is so effective in controlling heavy vaginal bleeding (menorrhagia) its use may eradicate the need for surgical procedures such as hysterectomy and removal by laser of the endometrium, with all their potential complications.

One concern has been the possible effect such a device may have on cervical cell cytology. Studies have been reassuring in showing that no cell changes have been found when compared with women using an intra-uterine contraceptive device (IUCD) over six years.

Also reassuring is the fact that in the 10,000 women-years of study no harmful effects were observed in the cardiovascular, liver or metabolic systems. Mirena offers a significant advance in contraception.

The LNG IUD may eventually be used as a possible source of the progestogen for endometrial protection used by women in association with menopausal oestrogen replacement therapy.

Unipath personal contraceptive system (UPCS)

This recently introduced product is a hand-held monitor that stores information about a woman's menstrual cycle. Eight urine stick tests are taken each month, and the colour code of the monitor (red, amber or green) indicates fertile or non-fertile days. The method, therefore, may be used for contraception, or for planning a family. For further information see address section.

Non-hormonal contraception

Spermicide and barrier methods

This group includes condoms, diaphragms and cervical caps. Condoms often have a spermicidal lubricant. With a diaphragm or cervical cap a spermicide has to be used before fitting, both to assist fitting and to improve the barrier effect. Diaphragms may be ineffective and difficult to use if there is any degree of prolapse, but the arch-spring variety and the vimule suction cervical cap can be effective.

Barrier methods are more effective for older women in the main, partly because their fertility is declining but also because they are more experienced in, and careful about, using contraception.

Spermicides
Currently all vaginal spermicides used in the UK employ detergents (surfactants) as their active ingredient; 80 per cent of all of them contain nonoxynol-9, which is altered to produce the same acidity level as the vagina; the remaining 20 per cent use either octoxynol or Di-isobutylphenoxypolyethoxyethanol as their spermicide. They work by causing disintegration of the sperm through 'membrane disruption'.

Types of spermicide currently available are:

Spermicide type	Active constituent
Delfen Foam	5% nonoxynol-9
Ortho Creme	2% nonoxynol-9
Duracreme	2% nonoxynol-9
Duragel	2% nonoxynol-9
Ortho Gynol Jelly	1% Di-isobutylphenoxy-polyethoxyethanol
Gynol II	2% nonoxynol-9
Staycept Jelly	1% octoxynol
Ortho Forms	5% nonoxynol-9
Staycept pessaries	6% nonoxynol-9
Double Check	6% nonoxynol-9
C Film	9.67 mg nonoxynol-9 on each square

There are some reports of vaginal irritation (stinging and burning) during and after spermicidal use, and occasionally infections of the Candida albicans variety (vaginal thrush) have been reported.

The suitability of another product, Chlorhexidine, as a vaginal contraceptive is being investigated. Its spermicidal activity is comparable to that of the surfactant spermicides but it does not act through membrane disruption and it is less sensitive than the former group to dilution by the vaginal and cervical mucus.

Barrier methods
Intra–uterine contraceptive device (IUCD or coil) The IUCD requires insertion by a doctor and usually needs to be changed every 3-5 years. It provides continuous protection against pregnancy, with a low failure rate (2 per cent, which is similar to that of a POP). IUCDs come in various shapes and sizes. Some are made entirely of plastic, while others contain copper.

When considering this form of contraception, certain disadvantages should be borne in mind: insertion may be painful; infection of the pelvic area can sometimes result from IUD usage; periods may be heavier, painful and/or last longer; the risk of ectopic pregnancy will be higher; and if there is a known metal allergy (for example, causing problems with rings and watches), the user may not be able to tolerate copper in the device.

Diaphragms and caps Diaphragms are thin rubber circular domes that are kept in place and shape by a rubber-covered metal rim. Caps are smaller and fit firmly over the cervix; they come in three forms, the vault, the cervical and the vimule. These devices are used in conjunction with a spermicidal jelly or cream. They may be inserted hours before intercourse and must remain in position for at least 6 hours afterwards. The failure rate is 2-5 per cent and there are no side effects.

Initial fitting must be done by a doctor or nurse to ensure the correct size.

These devices are worth considering by women who cannot use hormonal contraception and are prepared to accept a slightly lower level of protection. However, practice will help to achieve better contraception, as well as greater peace of mind. They are generally more suitable for women living with a partner.

Sponges Made of polyurethane foam impregnated with spermicide, these are 5 cm wide and have a small loop to assist removal. They can be purchased over the counter. One size fits all and the user can fit her own. However, the failure rate is 20-25 per cent, so these are more suitable for women over 40 whose fertility has begun to decline.

Condoms (male) Made of thin latex rubber and available either pre-lubricated (with spermicide or otherwise) or dry, these can be purchased over the counter. The condom is rolled on to the erect penis prior to any vaginal contact. There are no side effects, effectiveness is high with proper usage (but lower than that of the contraceptive pill), and some protection against sexually transmitted diseases, including AIDS, is provided. Where sexual union is infrequent, where medical history makes hormonal contraception inadvisable, and where the woman wishes her male partner to take responsibility for contraceptive protection, the condom is a viable option, and there is of course no need to consult a doctor or nurse before use.

Condoms (female) These are not a new concept. In 1920 a variety known as Capote Blanco was available by mail order, and Capote Anglaise, a similar product also known as Ladies' Own Sheath, was sold at surgical stores in the 1960s. In 1992 an improved version,

Femidon, was made available in the UK 'over the counter'. The open end of this loose-fitting, soft polyurethane sheath, 15 cm long, is attached to a flexible ring 7 cm in diameter. A firmer separate polyurethane ring measuring 6 cm in external diameter assists in insertion and anchoring the closed end into the upper vagina and around the cervix. The condom is supplied with silicone-based lubricant and is intended for single use only. Research so far shows that, on the plus side, it rarely splits during use; men experience less loss of sensitivity than they do with the 'male' condom; it provides protection against sexually transmitted diseases and greater protection than other barrier methods against viral infections, including HIV; and its failure rate is no higher than that of other condoms (15 per cent); moreover, its use is controlled by the woman herself, without the use of chemicals. The downside is that its insertion disrupts foreplay; its size and appearance are unappealing; its outer ring may cause discomfort or soreness; the inner ring may cause soreness to the partner; and it may feel cold and be slightly noisy in use.

Overall, however, it is a useful product which also provides protection against infection. For the older woman whose fertility is low during the transition years at the menopause it is a barrier contraceptive worth considering to bridge the gap between ceasing COC pills and not needing contraception at all.

Natural methods None of the following methods of birth control is recommended, as all are unreliable, but if religious beliefs, for example, prohibit all forms of contraceptive protection they may be better than nothing. Note that the effectiveness of the temperature and mucus evaluation methods depends on the female partner having regular cycles and being free of infection.

Temperature A graph is kept of the basal body temperature (taken rectally before getting out of bed each morning). When ovulation occurs, a sharp rise in temperature will be noticed. The raised temperature should continue for three days, after which begins the 'safe period', lasting until the next menstrual bleed.

Mucus evaluation Cervical mucus is evaluated daily. Ovulation occurs when the cervical mucus is at its most slippery and stretchable. The 'safe period' begins after the wet and slippery discharge ceases.

Coitus interruptus During intercourse, the penis is withdrawn from the vagina before ejaculation to prevent sperm entering the cervix. However, it is possible that sperm will be present at the tip of the erect penis prior to ejaculation. Moreover, whatever the intention before intercourse, it is likely that in the heat of the moment the penile withdrawal may not take place. Risk of pregnancy with this method is therefore high, as is the level of frustration felt by one or both partners through unfulfilled desire.

Sterilisation

The principle of sterilisation, of which hysterectomy (see Chapter 10) is an extreme form, is to disintegrate the Fallopian tubes so that the egg cannot be fertilised by sperm. As the ovaries are not touched, menstrual periods continue until the natural menopause. When ovulation occurs, the egg travels down the tube as far as is possible, then dies and gradually dissolves.

Sterilisation is a highly reliable form of contraception, and in both the UK and the USA it is the first choice of women over 35.

Whatever method of sterilisation is used, none will affect the menstrual cycle or the sex life. However, it is not recommended for women who have had a recent abnormal cervical smear or for those with any uterine or ovarian disorder.

Sterilisation must always be regarded as irreversible, because although, depending on which technique was used, a reversal operation might be possible, this is both complicated and prone to fail; moreover, there is no guarantee of conception subsequently.

The various types of sterilisation procedure are laparotomy, minilaparotomy, laparoscopy and vaginal sterilisation.

Laparotomy
Also known as tubal ligation (having the tubes tied), this is not a serious operation but it does require a general anaesthetic and a short stay in hospital. A small cut (5–8 cm) is made across the abdomen, usually just below the pubic hairline, the tubes are brought to the surface, each is tied in two places, and the short length of tube between the ties is removed.

Minilaparotomy

This is similar to a laparotomy, but the incision made is shorter. The uterus and tubes are pushed, by a special instrument inserted into the uterus from the vagina, towards the opening in the abdomen so that the tubes can be tied. This procedure can be carried out under local anaesthetic and is likely to cause less discomfort than a laparotomy.

Laparoscopy

A laparoscope (like a very narrow telescope) is inserted through a 1-cm cut just below the navel and a second cut made lower down to facilitate the tying of the tubes. This is the quickest and simplest method, usually performed under a local anaesthetic and likely to cause the least discomfort.

Vaginal sterilisation

Entry is via the vagina under general anaesthetic and the procedure is irreversible. This procedure is little used now.

All these types of sterilisation carry a small degree of risk, either from the general anaesthetic, if applicable, or from accidental damage to an organ or blood vessel during the operation. Subsequent complications are rare but could include bleeding, raised temperature, severe pain in the abdomen or uterus, and difficulty in urinating. Occasionally the ends of a tube may grow together again, bringing risk of pregnancy; about 10-20 per cent of such pregnancies turn out to be ectopic.

There is some evidence that the sterilisation procedure gives rise to heavier periods, and an increase in PMS symptoms of up to 30 per cent. These are thought to be due to an upset in the balance of ovarian oestrogen/progesterone hormones caused by nerve and prostaglandin alteration after tubal surgery, and alteration of blood supply. Research into this matter continues.

CHAPTER **9**

INCREASED HEALTH RISKS AT THE MENOPAUSE

THE MENOPAUSE brings not only increased risk of cardiovascular disease and osteoporosis, but also of breast cancer, endometriosis, ovarian disease and prolapse, among other disorders. Some of these may require surgery (see Chapter 10). However, the majority of women will experience few, if any, of these disorders.

Breast changes

The most common breast lumps are cysts, caused by retained fluid in a milk sac or duct, and fibroadenomas. The former are smooth but firm. The latter are solid, caused by overgrowth of fibrous and glandular tissue which knots together. Both types are benign. Other lumps, which may be cancerous, may feel the same on examination.

Formation of breast cysts is stimulated by methylxanthine, which is found in coffee, tea, cola drinks and chocolate. Cysts are more common in smokers, as nicotine also contains methylxanthine. Some women have found that taking evening primrose oil reduces the number of cysts they develop. Vitamin B6 (50 mg daily) and vitamin E (400 iu daily) have also been found helpful.

Women at increased risk of developing breast cancer are those who:
- already have cancer, especially of the ovary, colon, uterus or the other breast
- have menstruated for 35 years or more (those still having normal periods into the fifth decade would fall into this class)
- have a close female relative (mother, sister, aunt) with breast cancer
- have had no children or bore their first child after the age of 30

- are known to have 'benign breast change' (also called fibrocystic disease) or who have confirmed breast cysts or fibroadenomas. Benign breast change affects well over 30 per cent of women during the reproductive years. It reduces after the menopause as oestrogen levels fall. The condition is characterised by multiple small cysts interspersed with mild fibrous thickening of the breast tissue. The cause is unknown but likely to be hormone-related.

Studies show that one in ten breast lumps is cancerous. However, although breast cancer has now become the most common of all female malignancies (with over 15,000 recorded deaths from breast cancer in the UK in 1989), 11 out of 12 women will never develop it.

Diagnostic methods such as mammography, ultrasonography and breast aspiration and needle biopsy enable any worrisome breast lump to be investigated and identified.

Irregular bleeding between periods

While irregular periods around the menopause are normal, irregular bleeding is not. Any bleeding between periods, after the menopause or after intercourse should be discussed with a doctor. Such bleeding requires investigation because it may indicate cancer in its early, and curable, stage.

Heavy regular periods

This distressing and common complaint around the menopause may lead to fatigue and anaemia, besides being inconvenient. The usual causes are natural hormone swings or fibroids; less likely is a cancerous growth. It is important to seek medical advice.

Abdominal pain or heaviness in the pelvis

Pain may be experienced both during periods and at other times. Painful periods, called dysmenorrhoea, are due to severe cramping of the muscle wall of the uterus as it expels its lining, the endometrium.

Prostaglandins (hormone-like substances produced from fatty acids) are present in most body cells. They are identified, like vitamins, by a numbered letter. Prostaglandins alter body chemistry and their influence is widespread, affecting such areas as the heart, intestine, blood vessels and uterus. It is known that prostaglandins of the F_{2a} and E_2 series are responsible for menstrual cramps. Anti-prostaglandin drugs have been developed to reduce their effects. Examples are mefenamic acid (Ponstan) and naproxen sodium (Synflex). These medications can ease troublesome menstrual cramps.

Abdominal pain that occurs when there is no period is likely to be caused by fibroids, endometriosis, ovarian disease or pelvic or urinary infection.

Fibroids

These are dense, fibrous growths which can occur within the uterine wall, outside the uterus or within its cavity, attached by a pedicle or stalk. However, they are more commonly found between the inner and outer walls of the uterus (see Figure 7). Fibroids rarely become cancerous. Over 50 per cent of women have fibroids of some size associated with the uterus.

As fibroids are oestrogen-dependent they tend to grow bigger during the fertile years but diminish after the menopause. The fluctuating, and often high, oestrogen blood levels of the peri-menopause may cause these fibrous bundles to enlarge at this phase of life, causing heavy periods, abdominal discomfort and pelvic heaviness. The use of HRT may also cause them to increase in size.

Examination by a doctor and pelvic ultrasonography can confirm the diagnosis.

Endometriosis

In this painful condition cells of the endometrium migrate, possibly propelled by reverse Fallopian tube contractions, to surrounding pelvic organ surfaces. Common sites for endometriosis formation are the lining wall of the pelvic area, supporting ligaments, outer walls of the Fallopian tubes, ovaries, bowel and bladder. Sometimes fragments of endometrial tissue embed themselves in the muscle wall of the uterus itself, a condition known as **adenomyosis**. As the endometrial cells are under the influence of ovarian hormones they bleed cyclically, causing severe pain at times and producing adhesions, which fix one pelvic organ to another with tight fibrous

143

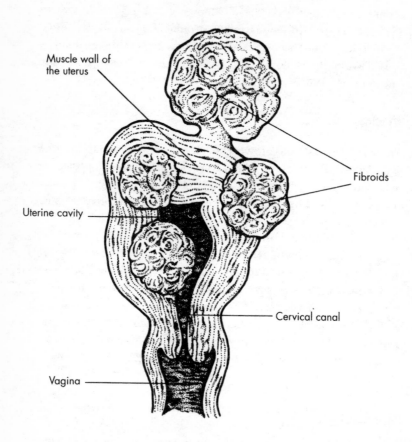

Figure 7   Position of fibroids in relation to the uterus

bands. Infertility is common in women with this condition because the Fallopian tubes may become blocked. Intercourse is painful due to movement of the cervix or pressure on the vaginal wall from transplanted endometrial tissue nodules.

If after looking at the patient's medical history and performing a pelvic examination the medical adviser suspects endometriosis, he or she can arrange a laparoscopy (see page 139) to provide confirmation.

Among the medications that are useful in controlling the condition are danazol (Danol) and dydrogesterone (Duphaston). New gonadotrophin-releasing hormone drugs are being developed and may be used in the short term, but side effects are common. Surgical treatment may eventually be required. If endometriosis is successfully managed, concurrent HRT usage is not completely ruled out. However, very careful monitoring is required.

Ovarian disease

Any swelling of, or pain in, the lower abdomen should be reported to a doctor. Some ovarian cysts are malignant. Cancer of the ovary can spread quite rapidly and may give few early clues as to its presence. Transvaginal ultrasonography of the ovaries and pelvis can assist diagnosis; the newer technique of measuring CA125 serum antigen blood levels is being developed, as are methods to detect increased blood flow through the ovaries themselves. These screening techniques will provide better detection in the early stages when signs of disease are not readily apparent, and allow for more rapid treatment.

Taking combined oral contraceptives (COCs) in the later fertile years before the menopause will give significant protection against ovarian and endometrial cancer without increasing the risk of breast cancer.

A hormonal disorder known as polycystic ovarian syndrome (Stein Levinthal syndrome) can be the cause of irregular periods as well as being ultimately responsible for cystic enlargement of both ovaries. This condition is usually seen in younger women, but can occasionally be the cause of irregular periods in women in their late thirties and early forties, giving the impression of an early menopause.

In this disorder the chosen ovarian follicle does not fully mature and rupture. Instead, it is trapped below the surface of the ovary.

Consequently, ovulation does not take place and the pituitary gland continues to produce follicle-stimulating hormone in ever-greater quantities in an effort to trigger the release of an egg. As a result of this more and more follicles are stimulated and become trapped. Over some months the surface of the ovary becomes studded with unripened and unruptured cysts. The ovaries increase in size and become polycystic.

While it is normal for adrenal glands and ovaries to produce some male hormone (testosterone), women with polycystic ovarian syndrome, because of the enlargement of their ovaries, produce extra testosterone. Higher than normal blood testosterone levels often cause hirsutism, the abnormal growth of dark, coarse, facial and body hair. This usually appears quite rapidly, and should not be confused with the fuzzy hair that many women have on their upper lip.

Polycystic ovarian syndrome can be controlled by hormonal therapy; surgery may however be required as well.

Prolapse of the uterus

The supporting ligaments of the uterus and vagina, which may have been stretched by childbirth, become weaker as the menopause is approached. The dwindling supply of oestrogen in the menopausal years also reduces the elasticity and firmness of tissue and skin, allowing the uterus to descend into the mid and lower vagina. Varying degrees of prolapse are thus produced. A loose pouch of vaginal skin, like an inverted pocket, with the bladder attached, may protrude into the cavity of the vagina: this is a **cystocele.** A similar prolapse of the bowel and back wall of the vagina is called a **rectocele**. Either condition, if severe, may require corrective surgery, in the form of an anterior or posterior repair (see Chapter 10).

Stress and urge incontinence

A cystocele and to a lesser extent a rectocele may give rise to poor bladder control causing a sudden desire to pass urine (urge syndrome) or leakage of small amounts or urine when coughing, sneezing or running (stress incontinence). Surgical correction by colporrhaphy may be required.

The skin lining the vagina and urethra has the largest

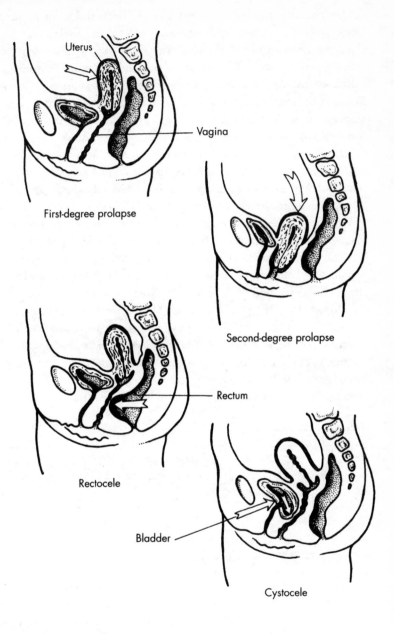

Figure 8   Prolapses, rectocele and cystocele

concentration of oestrogen receptors in the body and is, therefore, highly sensitive to changes in oestrogen levels. At the menopause the bladder muscle (trigone) atrophies. The blood supply to the vagina reduces, which causes thinning of its wall and makes inflammation, infection and ulceration more likely. The urethra shortens, which increases the risk of infection, and becomes narrower, which in turn leads to more frequent, and painful, urination and urgency (the 'urethral syndrome', see page 152).

In the absence of a cystocele or rectocele, stress incontinence often responds to a combined treatment regime of vaginal estriol (1 mg per day) and oral phenylpropanolamine (an alpha adrenergic agonist) 50 mg twice daily.

Urge incontinence is usually due to either sensory urgency or bladder muscle weakness. The former is caused by increased sensitivity to urinary bladder filling,while the latter is related to weakness of bladder and urethral muscle walls. Both form part of the 'urge syndrome' and both may be assisted by a series of exercises developed by Dr Arnold Kegel. These involve isolating and strengthening the sphincter muscle (pubo–coccygeus), which controls urination. If the tightening and relaxing of this muscle is routinely practised (an exercise that can be done at any time, anywhere), it will not only help to overcome the incontinence but will also strengthen the muscles used in sexual intercourse.

Table 20: Kegel exercises

To locate your sphincter muscle, simply stop the flow of urine while urinating; this is contraction of the sphincter muscle. Practise a few times, stopping and starting at will.

The routine

Three and one:

Contract your sphincter muscle for three full seconds, then release for one second. Repeat six times, three times daily for a few days. Then repeat 12 times a day for a week.

OR

One and one:

Contract your sphincter muscle strongly for one second and release for one second. Repeat 20 times, three times per day. Speed up the contractions so that you experience a 'fluttering' feeling.

OR

Ten and five:
Contract the sphincter muscle for ten full seconds (this will take practice). Relax for five seconds. Repeat five times, three times a day.

In addition sensory urgency appears to respond beneficially to vaginal treatment with oestrogen in the form of Vagifem pessaries (17B oestradiol 25 mcg pessaries) – 1 or 2 daily for 2-3 months.

Vaginal and urinary infections

Infections of both the vagina and the urinary tract may occur at any time of life, but because the lining walls of these areas tend to become thin at the menopause susceptibility to infection is increased.

The immune system, which protects and defends against infection, is directly influenced by the level of oestrogen and progesterone in the body. Research being undertaken at Guy's Hospital, London suggests that women who undergo surgical procedures during a certain phase in their menstrual cycle are more likely to have a favourable outcome. This 'cycle' timing of a surgical procedure indicates that hormone levels can influence the immune system. The defence mechanism also embraces the white blood cells, especially the macrophages and lymphocytes in the form of their B- and T-cells. Macrophages release prostaglandins, which play a vital role in another body defence action, inflammation. Healthy lymphocytes, when triggered to act in defence, may produce from their B-cells certain immunoglobulins which protect against infection.

At the menopause the immune system and its various components may function less efficiently. Consequently, infection becomes more likely. If prostaglandin reduction, especially of the D_2 series, occurs this can lessen resistance to infection of the skin and mucous membrane areas. The vaginal acidity level may also fall due to reduced hormone presence, which in turn diminishes the protective effect of the acid-loving Döderleins bacillus in the vagina.

The application of the proprietary product Aci-Jel (0.9 per cent acetic acid jelly) intravaginally once or twice daily may help to prevent infection.

Vaginal infections

Some clear vaginal discharge is normal and usual. An increased amount of clear discharge all through the cycle is often found by women who use the oral contraceptive pill. An increase at ovulation time only is commonly reported by women not taking the pill. Both situations are normal. Any blood-stained discharge should, however, be reported to a doctor.

An infected discharge is often coloured, perhaps yellow/green, and sometimes frothy. A thick, cream-cheese consistency is frequently found with yeast/fungal infections. Do not attempt home remedies – always consult a doctor. The delicate genital and urinary tract membranes require professional care.

Infections of the vagina are caused by a variety of organisms, many of which are sexually transmitted. Examples are:

Trichomonas vaginalis (TV), a protozoa organism which produces a copious, watery, yellow/green malodorous discharge. Its origins are obscure, but 60–80 per cent of male partners of infected women unknowingly harbour the organism in their urinary tract. It can therefore be passed back and forth through sexual intercourse, with the male having little sign apart, perhaps, from slight burning after ejaculation.

Metronidazole (Flagyl) tablets and pessaries are an effective treatment. It is important that any sexual partner should also be treated. Alcohol should be avoided during a course of metronidazole as it can cause an unpleasant reaction.

Hemophilus vaginalis (HV), sometimes called gardnerella, is a bacterium. It produces a grey-white discharge with an offensive fishy odour. Ampicillin (Penbritin) is effective in treatment and a five- or six-day course is usually sufficient. Metronidazole is also effective in a dosage of 400 mg twice daily by mouth for one week or a single dose of 2 g.

E coli infections can also occur in the vagina, but are more common in the urinary tract. Response to Ampicillin is rapid.

Candida albicans is a normal inhabitant of the body and of the vagina in 40 per cent of women. Vaginal fungal infection is often called candida, moniliasis or thrush. If the acidity level falls in the area where the candida is present the resulting increased alkalinity encourages its growth. The following factors are known to create this opportunity: pregnancy; oral contraceptive usage (but less so with lower-dosage preparations); diabetes; increased blood sugar levels; use of antibiotics; and increased stress and tension.

Severe itching with redness and swelling of the affected area can result. A thick, white, curdlike vaginal discharge easily spreads the infection to the rectal area and inner thighs. Any sexual partner is likely to be quickly infected, and the candida can rapidly spread beneath the foreskin of the penis. Both sexual partners must use medication, and treatment may sometimes extend from three to five weeks, the candida being stubborn to eradicate.

Both Diflucan and Sporanox are taken by mouth; they are usually used only when satisfactory results have not been achieved with the locally-applied preparations, because they are more potent.

It is possible that more than one infection may be present at the same time. To check, a 'culture and sensitivity' test is made of the offending discharge. A swab is taken and if an organism is found to be present on the culture, appropriate medication can be prescribed.

Two groups of especially effective genital antifungal medications are:

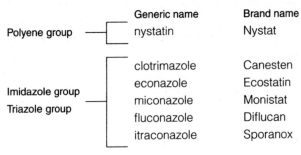

	Generic name	Brand name
Polyene group	nystatin	Nystat
Imidazole group	clotrimazole	Canesten
	econazole	Ecostatin
	miconazole	Monistat
Triazole group	fluconazole	Diflucan
	itraconazole	Sporanox

Many vaginal infections referred to nowadays as sexually transmitted diseases may not be caused by sexual contact. Many women who succumb to vaginal and urinary infections have no sexual partner. Vaginal infections also occur quite commonly after childbirth.

151

Sexually transmitted disease (STD)

Examples of diseases transmitted by sexual contact include gonorrhoea and syphilis.

Gonorrhoea, with an incubation period of two to seven days, is the most prevalent communicable disease in the USA (and in Europe generally), where over one million cases are reported each year. The organism may affect the urethra, cervix, rectum and vaginal passage. Complications, which can be serious, include abscess formation, pelvic inflammatory disease and infertility.

If you notice a yellow or blood-stained discharge, see your doctor at once, or attend a special STD clinic.

Syphilis, the most serious of all sexually transmitted diseases (apart from AIDS), is again on the increase, according to the number of reported cases. Early symptoms, such as a small sore, may disappear spontaneously, yet years later the disease can return, with devastating consequences in 30 per cent of all untreated cases. The disease is highly infectious, with an incubation period of 10-90 days following exposure, three weeks being the average. The infecting organism is the corkscrew-shaped Treponema pallidum. The usual first sign is a sore or chancre which may disappear but more usually increases in size and may within a week be as large as a marble. Immediate medical treatment is required, either by the GP or through the local STD clinic.

Young women in particular are at high risk of HIV infection. The World Health Organisation in Geneva reported in February 1995 that women represent half of all new HIV infections. Over 8 million women worldwide are now infected.

Urethral syndrome

It is not unusual for urinary and vaginal infections to be present together. It is possible that cross-infection between vagina and urinary tract is one cause of 'urethral syndrome'.

Common organisms infecting the urinary tract are E. coli; Proteus mirabilis; Staphylococcus saprophyticus; Chlamydia trachomatis; Trichomonas vaginalis; and Haemophilus vaginalis.

Symptoms of painful urination accompanied by frequency are often wrongly attributed to **cystitis** (inflammation of the bladder). In

50 per cent of women complaining of such symptoms, no bacteria can be found in the urine. The most common cause of the discomfort and frequency is **vaginitis** (inflammation of the vagina), but once this has been cleared up by appropriate treatment the urinary symptoms abate.

If no bacteria are found in the urine or vagina during examination the treatment should not be an antibiotic but an oestrogen cream applied to the urethral and vaginal openings two or three times daily for a week on a trial basis. A follow-up visit to the doctor for re-evaluation should then be made.

The clue to look for in urethral syndrome is an external rather than an internal sensation of discomfort on passing urine. Pain on urinating may be the result of dryness and cracking of the thinned and sensitive skin of the urethral tube which takes the urine from the bladder to the outside. This is common in women who are post-menopausal and lacking oestrogen.

Oestrogen cream preparations available for vaginal use include Premarin vaginal cream (natural conjugated oestrogens) and Dienoestrol vaginal cream (synthetic oestrogen).

Infections of the cervix

Sexual behaviour and infections of the cervix are linked. It is known that vaginal infections of the protozoa and bacterial variety which cause vaginitis can also cause **cervicitis** (inflammation of the cervix). In recent years there has been much research into the relationship between viral infections which are sexually transmitted, including herpes simplex virus II (HSV II) and human papillomavirus (HPV). These virus groups not only produce local infections but may also cause cell changes which can lead to cancer. HSV II is not thought to produce direct changes in the cells of the cervix but rather acts as a co-factor, thus allowing HPV to produce the cervical cell change in already weakened tissue.

Genital warts are believed to be caused by human papillomaviruses and to be sexually transmitted. HPV invades cells of the skin, in particular those of the surface, or squamous epithelium. It settles in the cell nucleus and can remain dormant for many years. There are over 60 types of HPV, each formed of strands of DNA (the acid carrying genetic information), and each numbered in order of discovery. Some types produce non-malignant cell changes, but others are responsible for pre-malignant and malignant change in areas of the female lower genital tract. As the virus spreads it produces warts which may be visible on the outer genitals and around the anal area. Internal lesions on the vaginal walls and cervix also occur. HPV types 16 and 18 are particularly virulent, with 50 per cent of invasive adenocarcinomas of the cervical canal showing the presence of one or other type. HPV6 and 11 are found more often in association with low-grade cervical cell changes and in condylomata (vaginal, anal and penile warts). Fifty per cent of male partners of women with condylomata have visible skin lesions. Between 2 and 5 per cent of women in today's sexually permissive society have HPV infection of the cervix.

Examination of the vulva and rectal area after application of 3-5 per cent acetic acid (vinegar) will identify whitish areas representing HPV presence. The area around the anus is quite commonly affected, although this does not always signify anoreceptive sexual activity. The degree of 'acetowhite' changes and 'sharpness' of the lesion margin indicates the degree of cell change present.

HPV detection is associated with a ten-fold or greater risk of cervical intraepithelial neoplasia (CIN) (see Chapter 11) compared to no infection. Women with HPV 16 or 18 are more likely to develop more serious CIN compared to women with lower-grade forms of HPV infection. HPV 16 is the most common form associated with surface cervical cancer, while HPV 18 is most common in cancer linked with the cervical canal and nerve- and hormone-associated tissue. It carries an increased risk of fatality, and is more invasive.

Prevention can most easily be achieved by maintaining a monogamous sexual relationship, but failing that latex condoms are the next best thing. A yearly cervical smear test (PAP smear) is strongly advised for all sexually active women.

Smoking is a risk factor, because carcinogens (substances which encourage cancer change) in tobacco smoke are thought to be directly secreted by cervical surface cells. Cervical cancer kills 2,000 women each year in Britain, and of those affected *most have never had a cervical smear test* (see Chapter 11).

Treatment options depend upon the DNA type of the human papillomavirus and the location of the disease. They include:

Cryosurgery   Liquid nitrogen, carbon dioxide or nitrous oxide is applied to the cancerous cells at a temperature of -89°C (or lower).

Electrocautery   An electric spark is applied to the cancerous cells to evaporate cell water and cause tissue destruction.

Laser surgery   This destroys tissue by vaporising it with a CO_2 laser beam.

Topical preparations   For vulval, peri-anal and penile warts, trichloracetic and bichloracetic acid or 5-fluorouracil can be applied directly to the skin using a small brush or cotton-tipped applicator. Podophyllin 25 per cent in tincture of benzoin is now being used less, but a purified form of the active ingredient podofilox has successfully completed trials in the USA and may be available in the UK soon as Podofilox 0.5 per cent topical skin solution. Topical treatments are painless and take only a few minutes. A further application in one week is usual.

Interferon therapy   Substances called interferons are produced when lymphocytes, fibroblasts or macrophages are activated to enhance their immune action. The interferons are capable of 'interfering' with viral multiplication, thus causing an antiviral action within the tissue cell which has been attacked, making replication and growth of the virus impossible. Interferon can be painted directly upon the tissue affected (vaginal, anal or cervical warts, for example) or injected – either into a muscle in the hip or arm or directly into the affected area. Side effects may include raised temperature, chills, headache, diarrhoea and nausea. When interferon therapy is used alone treatment results are only fair, but they are better when it is used in combination with other topical chemicals and surgical procedures (as described above).

Combined therapy   Combinations of different treatments have been effective in the management of HPV infections, which may be difficult to eradicate with one regimen alone. Examples of combined therapies are cryosurgery and CO_2 laser surgery – cervical intraepithelial neoplasia (CIN) – for cervical cancer; CO_2 laser surgery and 5-fluorouracil – vaginal intraepithelial neoplasia (VAIN)

– for vaginal cancer; and CO_2 laser surgery and local excision – vulvar intraepithelial neoplasia (VIN) – for vulval cancer. Follow-up smear tests are important. Many CIN lesions clear up completely but should be carefully monitored by six-monthly smear tests.

The future

Attempts are under way to develop a vaccine to protect against HPV infections responsible for increased risk of cervical cancer. This would reduce the number of cases, which increase each year by 5,000 in the UK and by 500,000 worldwide. This viral vaccine could be given to all children before puberty to give general HPV protection. Such a vaccine might also act as a booster to the immune system, and could be given to women who show early signs of cervical cell change.

At present, however, women with HPV infection should be aware that the disease cannot always be cured.

CHAPTER 10

COMMON SURGICAL PROCEDURES

No surgical procedure is unique to the menopause, but there are certain operations which menopausal women should know about.

Of the ten most commonly performed operations in North America, four are conducted on women. The percentage of women undergoing the same operation varies from country to country – for example, 12 per cent of British women undergo hysterectomies, compared with 25-30 per cent in the USA, Canada and Australia. Today, with newer treatments available, some surgical operations can be modified and others avoided entirely. It is important, therefore, that any proposed operation, and the possibility of alternative treatment, is fully discussed with the general practitioner. It is also advisable to talk to the surgeon.

There is no reason why you should not ask for a second opinion before agreeing to a major surgical procedure, or any operation for that matter, if you are at all in doubt or if you feel you have not been given adequate information.

Prior to any surgical procedure taking place the patient is asked to sign a consent form. Before signing, be sure that you have asked the following questions:

- What is the reason for the operation?
- What is going to be done?
- Who will perform the operation?
- How long will I be in hospital?
- How long will recovery take?
- Are there likely to be any permanent after-effects?
- Will I be sterile, and could my sex life be affected?

Breast biopsy

Fibrocystic breast disease (benign breast disease) is common, occurring in 30 per cent of all women. It is less usual, however, after the menopause. The cause is unknown. The condition takes the form of multiple small cysts interspersed with fibrous thickening, causing lumpiness and tenderness, which may increase premenstrually. Occasionally a single cyst enlarges and forms a distinct lump. The presence of any lump or mass requires investigation. Until recently a surgeon would routinely remove this lump by excision, but it is now common practice to use a needle to drain the lump of any fluid, thereby establishing a diagnosis. This 'aspiration procedure' has progressed further, and two modified techniques have been developed: the Mammotest and the Bard Monopty gun. Both methods allow tissue from a suspicious lump to be sucked up a fine-bored needle for accurate examination and diagnosis under the microscope.

Techniques are now available for accurate placement of a fine needle for aspiration biopsy into a lesion identified by mammography but which may be so small that it cannot be felt during breast examination. One is stereotactic radiography, another sonar mammography. Both allow a needle to be guided into a cyst or solid lesion to obtain fluid or cell material for cytological assessment. Unnecessary open surgery may thus be avoided.

Advancement in breast X-rays (mammography) and how these help identify very early breast cancer is discussed in Chapter 11.

Dilatation and curettage (D&C)

In this procedure the canal of the cervix is stretched, under a general anaesthetic, using a dilator. A curette, shaped like a small spoon on a long handle, is then carefully inserted into the cavity of the uterus. The endometrium, or lining, is scraped off by the curette and the tissue sample is sent to the laboratory for cell examination.

D&C is often advised if there is heavy or irregular vaginal bleeding. It is essentially a diagnostic procedure but may, however, be required following a miscarriage to reduce excessive bleeding, in which case it is curative. Following a diagnostic D&C patients usually leave hospital the same day.

A useful technique is now available which can reduce the frequency of unnecessary D&Cs. Sterile saline solution is introduced slowly into the cavity of the uterus by means of a catheter, causing it to distend. A vaginal probe is then introduced into the upper end of the vagina. This intra-vaginal ultrasound technique gives excellent pictures of the lining wall of the uterine cavity, and in particular the thickness of the wall (endometrium) and any distortion of it. Polyps may be distinguished from submucous fibroids and suction sampling of the endometrial cells obtained for cytology examination. This sonohysterogram procedure is useful for assisting in the diagnosis of unexplained uterine bleeding in the peri-menopausal years.

Endometrial biopsy

An experienced doctor can perform this procedure without an anaesthetic in the hospital out-patient department or in the consulting room. The tissue sample obtained, while not as large as from a D&C, can indicate any cell changes in the endometrium. It should be remembered that since only a small area of the endometrium is sampled, abnormal cells may be missed. This technique is useful, however, for evaluating abnormal vaginal bleeding which may occur in women taking HRT.

Trans-cervical endometrial resection (TCER)

Menorrhagia (heavy menstrual bleeding) is more common after the mid-thirties. It is often associated with hormone imbalance, or the presence of fibroids, which tend to enlarge the cavity of the uterus and increase the bleeding surface of the endometrium. Drug therapy may be helpful, although a hysterectomy (removal of the uterus) is frequently advised if other efforts fail.

Trans-cervical endometrial resection (TCER) is a new technique, developed in the USA and now being performed in some teaching hospitals in the UK. The John Radcliffe and Churchill Hospitals in Oxford, and the Royal Free Hospital in London, offer TCER to screened women with menstrual disorders. This procedure should be performed only by surgeons who have had special training in its use and considerable experience in its application. It is thought that

TCER could reduce the number of hysterectomies performed for menstrual disorders (see under hysterectomy, below) by up to 75 per cent. The complication rate for abdominal hysterectomy, according to one UK study, is 42.8 per cent; two studies in the USA state even higher figures, of up to 50 per cent. TCER, in trained hands, seems to produce far fewer post-operative problems; the complication rate stated for Canada and the USA is only 5 per cent.

During TCER the lining of the uterus is cut away (resected) under a local anaesthetic using a laser beam. This laser ablation procedure takes about 15-20 minutes. However, if the abnormal uterine bleeding is caused by either pelvic inflammatory disease or fibroids which are situated in a particular area of the uterus this new procedure may not be appropriate.

Pregnancy following removal of the endometrium is extremely unlikely.

Women taking HRT who have undergone endometrial resection should continue to take a progestogen with the oestrogen. This will prevent any risk of hyperplasia of microscopic endometrial tissue that may remain in any part of the uterine wall following TCER.

Hysterectomy

In the UK 20,000 hysterectomies are performed each year. A hysterectomy always means removal of the entire uterus. Other adjacent structures, if diseased, may be removed in addition.

In a simple, complete or total hysterectomy the entire uterus and cervix are removed. In a radical hysterectomy the uterus, cervix, tubes, ovaries and pelvic lymph glands are removed; this operation is performed in the treatment of certain pelvic malignancies. For a partial hysterectomy (rarely performed nowadays), the uterus is removed but the cervix is left in place.

All the above procedures are carried out via an incision through the lower abdomen.

In a vaginal hysterectomy the uterus and cervix are removed via the vagina, which is a technically difficult procedure to perform when large fibroids are present, but is often carried out when a prolapse repair is also required.

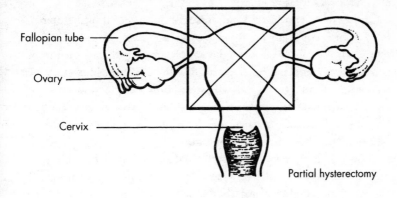

Fallopian tube

Ovary

Cervix

Partial hysterectomy

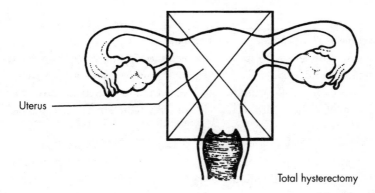

Uterus

Total hysterectomy

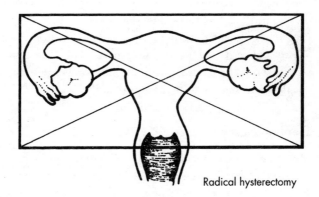

Radical hysterectomy

Figure 9   Different types of hysterectomy

Myomectomy

This is an alternative surgical procedure to a hysterectomy for treatment of certain fibroid tumours without removal of the uterus. It is more common in North America than in the UK. A myomectomy can be performed on any woman, provided the uterus is not heavily affected by fibrous growths. The procedure may be technically more difficult than a hysterectomy and blood loss may be greater. In peri-menopausal women endometriosis and fibroids often co-exist; a hysterectomy may be the more appropriate method of dealing with these combined conditions.

A new technique has been pioneered at the Royal Free Hospital in London whereby relatively large fibroids can be removed via the vagina, thus avoiding major abdominal surgery and reducing blood loss.

Removal of ovaries during hysterectomy

There is usually no reason for a woman to have her ovaries removed unless they are diseased – for example, by extensive endometriosis cysts or cancer. If both are removed an immediate menopause will begin; if only a part of one is conserved the menopause can be delayed.

Some gynaecologists, while performing a hysterectomy on women over the age of 40, still routinely remove perfectly normal ovaries. There is little justification for the removal of healthy ovaries on the pretext that they may one day become cancerous; the incidence of ovarian cancer in the UK is only 17 in 100,000 women each year. By comparison, 29 women out of every 100,000 who are pregnant will die from complications of childbirth or pregnancy.

Any concerns the patient may have about the removal of the ovaries should be discussed with the surgeon beforehand, to establish clearly what is going to be removed and why.

Oöphorectomy

It may be advisable for the ovaries to be removed (oöphorectomy) at the time of hysterectomy in the case of a pre-menopausal woman whose uterus is being removed owing to cervical cancer. Even where the ovaries are retained, they cease to function in 25-30 per cent of women within three to five years. Benign forms of ovarian

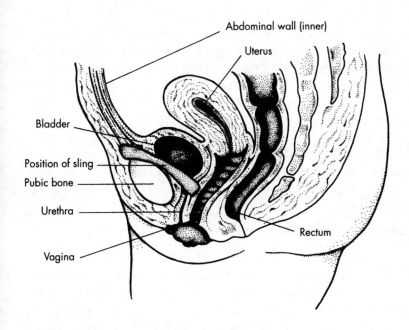

Figure 10   Colporrhaphy

disease (cysts) occur in approximately 8 per cent, and ovarian cancer is likely in 1.5 per cent.

In women aged 50 or more who have gynaecological surgery, prophylactic (precautionary) removal of the ovaries would reduce subsequent incidence of ovarian cancer by 11 per cent. In the younger woman for whom hysterectomy is advised because of non-cancer-related conditions, such as prolapse, fibroids or severe dysmenorrhoea (period pains), and the ovaries are found to be healthy at the time of surgery, the case for prophylactic oöphorectomy is weak and questionable. HRT would, however, be required, entailing medication, visits to the doctor to tailor the medication and repeat prescriptions. Moreover, ovarian removal may have a psychological effect, lending credence to the expression 'always a patient, never a woman'.

There may be circumstances, however, when removal of one or both ovaries is considered prudent, for example, recurrent or present ovarian cysts, endometriosis or severe and uncontrollable PMS.

Woman are strongly advised to heed the recommendations given at the beginning of this chapter before signing a consent form for surgery.

Anterior and posterior vaginal repair

If symptoms from either a cystocele or a rectocele are severe enough to cause discomfort or inconvenience, operative correction may be required. This is a form of plastic surgery which repairs the defect in the underlying muscles and connective supporting tissue of the anterior (front) or posterior (back) vaginal walls. At the same time a slack vagina can be restructured.

Colporrhaphy

In Chapter 9 the role of Kegel (pelvic) exercises in the improvement of urge incontinence was described. Stress incontinence, however, may require colporrhaphy. This surgical operation tightens the neck of the bladder and at the same time supports it. Any loose skin causing pouting and laxity of the vaginal wall can also be removed. On occasion, a sling is fashioned from surrounding body tissue to support the bladder base and the urethra (the tube conveying urine from the bladder to the outside). The Manchester-type repair is similar but also involves removal of the cervix and is little performed nowadays.

A newer procedure, the colposuspension, is increasingly used in suitable stress incontinence cases.

Cholecystectomy

Cholecystectomy (removal of the gall bladder) is more common, by a ratio of three to one, in women than in men. Each year, in the UK, 87 women per 100,000 aged 40-49 have a cholecystectomy as a result of gall bladder disease. In women who take HRT that number rises to 218. It is known that COC pills also increase the risk of gall bladder disease.

The incidence of gall bladder disease may be lessened by avoiding fatty food, increasing fibre intake and controlling weight.

The risk for gall bladder patients of taking HRT needs to be carefully weighed against other benefits which HRT can produce. Many women have asymptomatic (silent) gallstones which may become larger only when HRT is started and then give rise to problems such as indigestion, gas, flatulence and pain.

The non-surgical treatment of gallstones is being developed using the Lithotripter, a technique which employs sound waves. Better results have so far been obtained when the procedure is used to pulverise stones in the kidney rather than in the gall bladder.

CHAPTER 11

MEDICAL EXAMINATIONS AND SCREENING

DURING all phases of a woman's life, any unfamiliar physiological changes should be reported to a doctor for examination and all routine screening appointments attended. Listed below are the examinations and screenings that most women are likely to experience.

Pelvic examination

Any problem of vaginal discharge can be investigated by taking a swab from the vagina, which is then sent to a laboratory for culture and probable miscroscopic examination. The result will indicate what treatment is required.

A diagnosis of uterine prolapse in association with a cystocele or rectocele (see Chapter 10) can be made by means of a pelvic examination. This examination may also arouse suspicions of the presence of fibroids, though it will not confirm them. The insertion of a speculum into the vagina allows the cervix to be viewed, with illumination. Internal examination allows a doctor to feel the size and tenderness of the ovaries as well as the position and shape of the uterus. During an internal examination the doctor places the other hand on the patient's abdomen and applies gentle pressure to aid in the assessment of the internal structures.

The cervix

The cervix is the lower part of the uterus. It lies at the top of the vagina and projects into it. Two types of cells are found in different areas on the skin of the cervix:

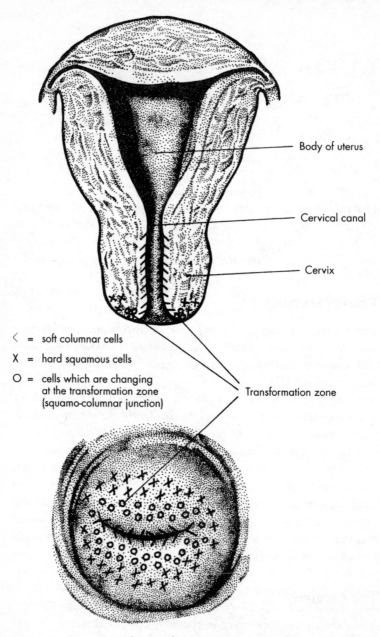

Body of uterus

Cervical canal

Cervix

〈 = soft columnar cells

X = hard squamous cells

O = cells which are changing
at the transformation zone
(squamo-columnar junction)

Transformation zone

Figure 11 The transformation zone

Columnar cells form a single tall layer of delicate mucous-producing cells which line the canal leading from the outer vaginal surface of the cervix and extend towards the inner uterine cavity.

Squamous cells are tougher, and form the multi-layered skin on the remainder of the surface of the cervix.

The point at which these two types of cell meet and merge into each other is called the squamo-columnar junction or the 'transformation zone'. (See Figure 11.)

Occasionally the columnar cells pout and thicken on the cervical surface. This 'erosion' is normal and happens frequently at times of increased hormone activity, for example, during adolescence, pregnancy, or with the use of the combined oral contraceptive pill.

Cervical smear (PAP smear)

In the 1930s the late Dr George N. Papanicolaou showed that cancer cells originating from the cervix and lining of the cavity of the uterus could be detected in the mucus of the vagina. Since then there have been many refinements in the way that cell material is collected, processed and interpreted. In recognition of his work, however, the term Papanicolaou smear, or PAP smear, has been retained.

To take a cervical smear, the doctor inserts a speculum into the vagina in order to see the cervix. The surface of the cervix is then gently scraped with a specially shaped spatula to gather cell material, which is placed on a labelled glass slide. The entrance to the cervical canal is also sampled, using an endocervical brush. A correctly taken cervical smear should contain cells from all three areas: the outer cervix (squamous cells), the cervical canal (columnar cells) and the 'transformation zone' (squamo-columnar junction). (See Figure 11.)

The glass slide is fixed in an alcohol solution and sent to a laboratory, where it is stained to show up the internal cell structure. A cytoscreener then examines the prepared slide and any abnormal findings are reported. In 1991 the British Society of Clinical Cytology (BSCC) asked all laboratories to record it in their reports if a smear was inadequate for accurate interpretation. Therefore, you should ask your doctor, when you receive your smear report, if the sample obtained was satisfactory *in all ways*. If the smear cannot be viewed clearly, the patient will be asked to attend for a repeat test.

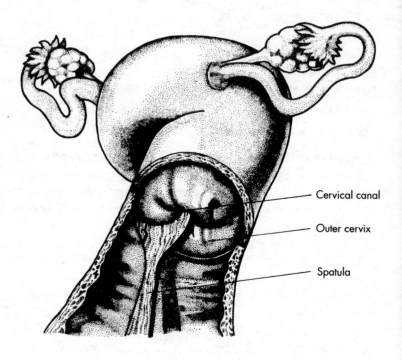

Cervical canal

Outer cervix

Spatula

Figure 12   Taking a cervical smear

Cervicography

Cervicography is a screening technique that has been used in the USA for several years for detecting abnormal cells on the cervix. It can be used in conjunction with a smear test to provide a more comprehensive evaluation of the cells of the surface of the cervix. It cannot, however, give evidence of the health of the cells in the cervical canal, or of the transformation zone if this area is deep within the cervical canal as often occurs in menopausal women. The use of the endocervical brush gives such evidence, however, and the combined usage of all these techniques provides complete screening cover.

The photographs (cervicograms) are taken after a vaginal speculum has been inserted and 5 per cent acetic acid has been applied to the cervix. The cervicograms are then projected on to a large screen for viewing. Occasionally the cervicogram may be out of focus, and a repeat visit necessary. The procedure can produce false alarms because the gynaecologist assessing the photographs will want to err on the side of caution if there is any suspicion of early cell change. Cervicography is not generally available, so it is advisable to continue with regular smear tests.

Cancer of the cervix

Cervical cancer usually starts at the transformation zone, where the delicate columnar cells merge and change to tougher squamous cells. Certain factors are thought to be responsible for its development. They are intercourse from an early age, frequent change of sexual partners, genital herpes, genital warts (human papillomavirus infection) and cigarette-smoking.

If the normal process of change at the transformation zone is altered by any of these factors an abnormal tissue change (dysplasia) takes place and this will produce an abnormal cervical smear result. The extent or degree of abnormal change reflects the severity and the potential risk of cancer developing. Dysplasia is now usually referred to as cervical intraepithelial neoplasia, or CIN. This term has replaced dysplasia when abnormalities are reported by the cytoscreener.

Table 21: Reporting of a cervical smear

HPV effects	HPV effects
slight dysplasia	CIN I
moderate dysplasia	CIN II
severe dysplasia } carcinoma-in-situ	CIN III

Key HPV – human papillomavirus
     CIN – cervical intraepithelial neoplasia

Abnormal smear test

When cells are seen on the smear test that suggest the presence of a pre-cancerous change, the smear test is abnormal. It is important to remember that there are degrees of change, and an abnormal smear test does *not* mean that cancer is present. However, it will mean that further investigation is required.

Vaginal infections may alter a smear result and the cytoscreener may then report an 'inflammatory' smear. In this case the doctor will prescribe appropriate medication and a repeat smear test will be given following treatment of the infection. If the repeat smear still shows CIN I or if any smear shows CIN II or III the patient will be referred to a gynaecologist for a colposcopic examination.

Colposcopy

This examination is very similar to a smear test. The cervix is exposed, then looked at by a colposcope, which is like a pair of binoculars with a spotlight. This low-powered microscope allows the viewer to recognise any abnormal cells on the cervix and to determine the degree of change. The instrument does not come into contact with the cervix, and under normal circumstances the procedure is painless and takes about 15 minutes.

Sometimes it is necessary to remove a small piece of tissue (a biopsy) for more detailed laboratory analysis by a pathologist, who will confirm the findings of the smear and colposcopy and determine whether there is any actual cancer cell change.

CIN (I, II and III) can be completely cured in 95 per cent of cases by the destruction of the abnormal cell area. The available methods of doing this are laser treatment, cryosurgery (freezing), electrodiathermy and cold 'coagulator'. All are equally effective (see Chapter 9).

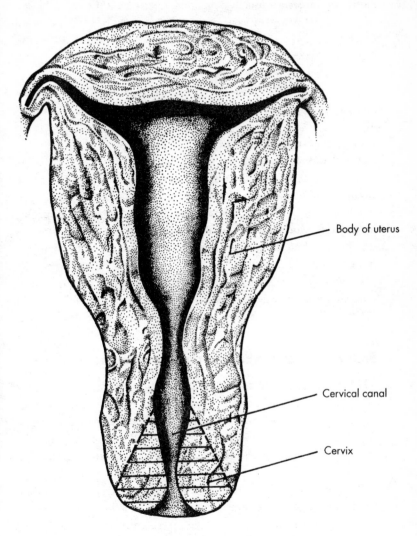

Body of uterus

Cervical canal

Cervix

Figure 13   Cone biopsy of cervix

Occasionally, abnormal tissue extends deeply into the cervical canal, in which case the colposcope may not view it. The aforementioned techniques cannot therefore be used, and a cone biopsy of the area is usually suggested. This entails the removal of a cone of tissue with the point of the cone extending into the cervical canal (see Figure 13). A general anaesthetic is required for this procedure, as well as a short stay in hospital.

After treatment, approximately 5 per cent of women will still show a form of CIN on follow-up examination. However, the great majority of these will respond very well to further repeat treatment.

Frequency of cervical smear tests

Cervical cancer is increasing. Every woman who is, or has been, sexually active should have regular smear tests, ideally every year up to the age of 65, and every two or three years thereafter.

Under the UK's present population cytology screening programme women are requested to attend for a smear test every three years. Any woman who wishes to have a more frequent test must have it done privately.

Obviously there are exceptions to this three-year rule for women who are (or previously have been) treated for CIN. In such cases the patient will be guided by her gynaecologist or family doctor.

Breast self-examination and breast awareness

This procedure may be carried out on the first few days following the end of the menstrual period. Women who no longer have periods can examine themselves on the first day of each calendar month. A chart should be kept and the date of each breast self-examination marked on it. Regular examination should alert women to any early change.

These are the changes that it should be possible to recognise: any difference in the size of one breast; one breast lower than the other; alteration in the position of the nipples; a breast lump or a local lumpy area; indrawing of a nipple; liquid escaping from a nipple; puckering or dimpling of the breast skin; a skin rash or change in texture or skin colour; enlarged glands in the armpits or above and below the collar bones; a swelling of the upper arm.

Figure 14 shows how to perform a breast self-examination.

If any changes in the breasts are found since the last examination, a doctor should be consulted at once. The chance that cancer is present is small, but it may take other tests to confirm this. It is also advisable for a doctor to examine the breasts once a year in addition to self-examination.

Cancer detection by this method is estimated at 26 per cent in all age groups, which indicates that many cancers are missed when compared to the 80–90 per cent sensitivity rate of mammography. In younger women the positive predictive value is lower, at about 4–6 per cent, which indicates that in women with positive findings the great majority do not have cancer. Additional benefit from breast self-examination may be gained by changing both attitude and frequency. Instead of examining the breasts every month as a ritual the exercise can be treated as part of life experience and grooming. Breast awareness allows women to become familiar with the feel and texture of normal breast tissue and the swings which can be perceived in it, as caused by monthly hormone changes or through age. Such *regular* breast examination has become known as breast awareness and may be carried out in conjuction with formal monthly examination as advised and shown by either the doctor or the practice nurse.

Mammography (breast X-ray)

Mammography reduces the death rate from breast cancer in women aged 50 and over. Each year in the UK there are 30,000 new cases of the disease and over 15,000 deaths from it. Of those women who develop breast cancer each year, half are over 65.

The death rate can be reduced by up to 40 per cent in women who attend for screening, the greatest benefit being in women of over 50. The incidence of the disease rises sharply with age: 80 per cent of all new cases and 88 per cent of all breast cancer deaths occur in women aged 50 and over.

Under current NHS policy women between 50 and 64 are invited for mammography, but those of 65 and over, among whom 50 per cent of the 30,000 new annual cases occur, receive no such invitation – a situation which should not be allowed to continue.

At the initial two-view screening 60 cancers are detected for every

How to look
Undressed to the waist, sit in front of a mirror in good light.

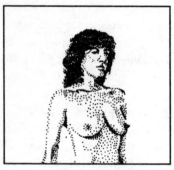

1. Look: hands at your sides or on your hips, look carefully at your breasts. Turn from side to side. Look underneath too.

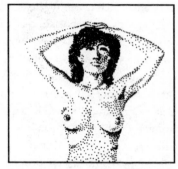

2. Lift: hands on your head, look for anything unusual, especially around the nipple.

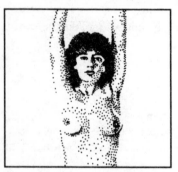

3. Stretch: arms stretched above your head, look again, particularly around the nipple.

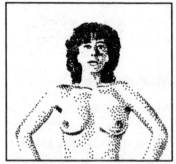

4. Press: hands on hips, press inwards until your chest muscles tighten. Look again, especially for any dimpling of the skin.

Figure 14   Breast examination

How to feel
Lie on a flat surface, head on a pillow, shoulder slightly raised by a folded towel.

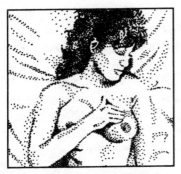

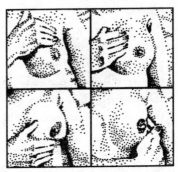

5. Left shoulder raised, feel the left breast with the right hand. Use the flat of the fingers, keeping them together.

6. Press the breast gently but firmly in towards the body. Work in a spiral, circling out from the nipple. Feel every part.

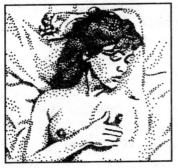

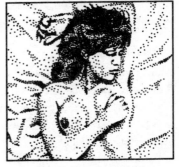

7. Left arm above your head, elbow bent, repeat the spiral carefully. Feel the outer part of the breast especially.

8. Finish by feeling the tail of the breast towards the armpit. Repeat all four stages on the other breast. Be thorough. Don't rush.

By kind permission of the Women's Nationwide Cancer Control Campaign.

10,000 women screened. At subsequent one-view screens about 35 cancers are identified for every 10,000 attending.

Up to 70 per cent of significant abnormalities detected by mammography cannot be felt upon examination, and these require accurate localisation by either ultra-sonography or stereotaxis to permit guided-needle aspiration cell biopsy (see Chapter 10) for definitive diagnosis.

Compared with cancers that can be readily felt, mammographically detected cancers are small and more likely to be non-invasive. Small invasive cancers are less likely than larger tumours to have spread to lymph glands and surrounding tissue.

Some 70-80 per cent of cancer detected by mammography may have a good prognosis. At initial screening where detection takes place, 20 per cent will be non-invasive (*in situ*), 20-25 per cent invasive and under 1 cm in diameter, and 25 per cent invasive and 1-2 cm in diameter.

To be life-saving, mammography must be efficient and women willing to comply with the treatment: in other words, there has to be a positive approach on both sides. Enthusiasm and encouragement from the GP, practice nurse and other medical personnel should produce higher compliance and attendance rates by patients to be screened, and greater confidence in its success.

The question of when screening should be started is controversial. Many radiologists feel it should begin between the ages of 35 and 40. This view is held by the American Cancer Society, the US National Cancer Institute and by both the American College of Radiology and the American Medical Association. Other groups, such as the American Colleges of Physicians and Obstetricians and Gynaecologists, the Canadian Task Force on Periodic Health Examinations and the Forrest Report (UK), feel that screening should be delayed until the age of 50. Numerous studies from around the world, including the Marks & Spencer Study in 1984 and a more recent UK study in 1988, have not settled the issue. (See the Bibliography for further references.)

The ideal frequency of mammographic screening has yet to be agreed. It is interesting that the incidence of cancer increases rapidly between years 2 and 3 after the initial screen, indicating that in women aged 50-64 a three-year gap is too long. The frequency may have to be reduced to 18-24 months. The British United Provident

Association (BUPA) advises that screening be started at 40 years and repeated every 12-18 months until age 50, then annually. There is evidence that the incidence of breast cancer is higher in older women. Suggestions have been made that screening should be continued until the age of 74, at repeat intervals under three years. The effectiveness of screening women younger than 50 has not as yet been proven. Age appears to be the only risk factor of sufficient value to influence routine screening policy at this time.

Breast density in women under 50 makes mammographic interpretation difficult, but with improved screening techniques, darker film production and improved high-technology equipment such as computerised imaging digital mammography (where hard-to-see breast areas are clarified by coloured rings) suspicious areas of tissue and minor flecks of calcium can be clarified. Small malignant cancers, of low harmful potential at this stage, can be spotted earlier before hazardous invasive disease occurs.

How safe is mammography?

There has been much media discussion recently about the safety of mammography, in view of the fact that it uses irradiation. One of the most up-to-date mammography screening units is the Siemens Mammomat-2. This machine is computer-controlled and automatically works out the lowest irradiation required to produce excellent-quality films. This is done by taking into consideration the breast density and thickness at each separate examination.

The amount of irradiation used for an initial two-film exposure on each breast is less than that received with a regular chest X-ray, or the irradiation a passenger is subjected to during a two-hour flight on Concorde. The risk is also no more than that attached to smoking half a cigarette. A subsequent mammography usually requires only one film view per breast, which means that the amount of irradiation is further reduced by one half.

The risk from a single-view mammogram in women aged 50 years or over may result in the occurrence of one extra breast cancer a year after ten years for every 2 million women screened.

Mammographic screening is the best method for detecting breast cancer. However, to be successful it requires highly trained radiologists to interpret the films, which need careful processing by expensive high-technology machinery.

Screening for colonic cancer

Colonic cancer is the second most common internal cancer in the USA. Fifteen per cent of cases occur in the 40-50 age group, and the overall incidence in the population is 45 per 100,000. It is now recommended that all individuals over 45 should have an annual occult blood (hidden blood) test, during which three stools are examined. This is a simple and painless procedure.

The best study to date, reported in 1988, was done in the Swedish town of Gothsburg and involved 27,700 subjects. Another large study, which has been in progress in Minnesota since 1980, should provide further collaborative information (see the Bibliography). Those who are at highest risk of colonic cancer are over 50 with a personal history of inflammatory bowel disease, polyps or ulcerative colitis.

The advisability of undergoing colonoscopy should also be discussed with the general practitioner if the patient falls into the higher-risk category and especially if there is a family history of cancer.

Genes have been isolated on chromosomes 17p and 18q which, if present, can help to predict the outlook for a patient with colorectal cancer. The genes on the two chromosomes probably influence the abnormal cell changes on the lining wall of the colon or rectum which produce tumour change.

CHAPTER 12

FIFTY YEARS ON – THE FUTURE

ADVANCES in technical and scientific expertise over the next five decades will make today's medical knowledge seem meagre. The human lifespan will be lengthened and new dietary regimes and stress management techniques will encourage activity, both physical and mental, well past the age of 90.

Genetics, nutrition and the human lifespan

Genetics is the study of heredity and the variation of inherited characteristics. Genes contain DNA, the chemical substance which transmits such characteristics from parent to offspring. The handing-down of this 'information' from an individual's parents determines several things: what a person will look like, how he or she will grow and whether he or she will inherit certain diseases or be resistant to others.

However, this is not the complete story. The way in which an individual develops is determined partly by genes but also by nutrition. Sound nutrition is the cornerstone of a healthy existence, and it is becoming clear that this must begin in the formative months of life, in the womb.

The future

In the future, if a woman (through better nutrition) is living to a greater age, she should expect her reproductive years to increase commensurately. Improved nutrition would also lead to her maturing and starting menstruation at an earlier age than nowadays.

A girl born in the year 2000 may be still fertile in her late fifties or sixties. Ovarian transplants, to avoid the menopause (which have to date been performed only on a few women), may be as commonplace in the future as oestrogen implants are now. An ovarian transplant combined with increased physical youthfulness may make pregnancy possible at 60 or 70. This new internal source of oestrogen and progesterone, from the ovary, will be more natural than any pill or patch. However, the eggs produced may or may not be the recipient's, depending on whether the transplanted ovary is her own or someone else's.

It is quite likely that within 50 years family organ banks will have been established. Members of a family will routinely leave their organs to be frozen for use by other members. (The risk of organ rejection at transplant is lessened when the donor organ comes from a family member.) Fatal accidents and other causes of violent death will be one source for the banks, but there will also be organs from those who will achieve longevity due to healthier lifestyles.

Young women who are to receive chemotherapy and/or radiation where the dosage is high enough to deplete the ovarian stock of follicles may in the future be able to have part of or a complete ovary removed as a preventive measure. These small follicles would be stored in bulk at low temperatures, thawed at the appropriate time and xenografted. Work on this procedure is currently taking place in Edinburgh.

In the future a lifespan of 110 years may not be a rarity. A woman who wishes to extend her years of fertility may decide to have one healthy ovary removed when she is in her thirties. This would be frozen and stored in a family organ bank for re-implantation when she is 60.

Those who have not committed an ovary to storage would still have the chance to receive a donor ovary from most teaching hospitals, where the organ would have been genetically typed for race, hereditary traits and blood grouping on receipt to make a suitable match for the recipient. Special traits of the donor would also have been carefully noted, with reference, for example, to intelligence, talents and other characteristics. A woman wanting an ovary for the purpose of pregnancy would therefore be able to select an organ which would produce eggs as genetically similar to her own as possible.

Pregnancy outside the womb

It is already possible for an egg to be taken at the time of ovulation, fertilised and placed in the uterus of a 'foster' mother, resulting in a normal pregnancy and the birth of a healthy child. An artificial uterus is now being designed which will be able to sustain the normal development of a human embryo to maturity at nine months. Whereas today's advanced neo-natal hospital units have facilities to care for infants who are premature by two or three months, an artificial uterus will make it possible for even younger infants to develop to the point where self-function can take over.

Screening out birth defects before conception

It is now possible to screen for genetic abnormalities before fertilisation of an egg by the sperm. This allows abnormal eggs, as opposed to embryos, to be rejected. Such analysis offers ethical and technical advantages over present methods, and will become even more sophisticated in the future. Genetic abnormalities for which screening can already be carried out include cystic fibrosis, haemophilia, hereditary blindness and genetic Huntington's chorea.

Pioneer work in this technique is taking place at St Mary's Hospital, London and in the USA, at the Masonic Hospital, Chicago and the University of Missouri.

The age of the gene hunter is here. Since the pioneering days of the mathematician and biologist Johann Mendel to the successes of Mark Lathrop and Jean Weissenbach, who have mapped the genome using microsatellite markers, finding the genes for human disease has become paramount. Complex diseases which involve more than one gene are the newest challenges in molecular genetics. The future, let us hope not too distant, should identify the genes responsible for mental illness, Alzheimer's, certain cancers, hypertension and asthma, to name a few. The possibilities for treatment and improvement in health are limitless as the gene hunt gains pace.

This, however, is far from being the end of the story. Gene medicine is just around the corner.

Gene medicine

This biotechnology targets genes at specific cells and then switches them on when they arrive. Research is concentrating upon a sophisticated guidance system using proteins to carry DNA into the nucleus of target cells where it mixes with the genes there. First, blood cells are removed from the body, the DNA targeting then takes place *outside* the body, and replacement by re-infusing follows. Clinical trials will soon take place, treatment of Gaucher's disease (splenic anaemia) being a likely initial candidate. The prospect of using the technique to protect the immune system of AIDS-sufferers from further attack by HIV is tantalising. Eventually the technique will be refined so that the process will be possible *within* the body, where it will be administered like any other medicine.

New horizons in contraception

It may not be too many years before the diaphragm, cap, IUCD and contraceptive pill are consigned to history as contraceptive methods.

It is now known that some women are infertile because their own immune system produces antibodies in response to their particular partner's sperm. The antibodies cause immobilisation and disintegration of the sperm, with resulting infertility.

An anti-sperm vaccine is being developed which will work on the same principle. When given to a woman, such a vaccine will destroy the sperm; in a man the vaccine will cause its immobilisation. Hormone production will be left unaltered, ovulation unimpeded, but pregnancy prevented.

Such a vaccine would be protection against pregnancy for x number of years or months dependent upon its strength. Reversal of action within four or six weeks would be possible by the use of an anti-sperm vaccine.

Advances in cancer diagnosis and treatment

Advances in the treatment of certain identified breast tumours are being pioneered in one of London's teaching hospitals. A high-powered laser beam is directed at the abnormal cells, destroying the malignancy without damaging surrounding tissue. This procedure is complemented at present by other established forms of cancer therapy. Prevention of breast cancer can, however, only be brought about when its cause is known.

A vaccine for certain forms of cervical cancer is under intense study. A link between certain viruses and cancer of the cervix is already known to exist.

Control of breast cancer by vaccine should become possible. Future research will investigate the fact that genetic abnormalities are present in some women with breast cancer.

Two cancer genes have been positively identified, and no doubt others will follow. A link between cancer risk and certain infective processes has been established, hepatitis viruses and liver cancer are associated, and Epstein Barr virus associated with nasopharangeal cancer risk in South East Asia. Epstein Barr virus also shares a relationship with Hodgkin's disease and possibly to other lymphomas and the leukaemias. It is now thought that some 10 per cent of human cancers may result from infective processes.

Genetic markers have been identified in sufferers of colonic cancer, the third most common cause of cancer death among women. Early screening is therefore of great importance. It should also be possible to diagnose ovarian cancer earlier, using similar techniques.

Screening methods already allow malignant cells to be 'tagged' with radioactive markers injected intravenously. This means that very early cancers can be detected and 'marked' using a nuclear magnetic imaging chamber in which the patient is slowly rotated.

The mind and physical disease

The relationship between the mind, the immune system and the prevention and control of illness has long been suspected and is likely to be confirmed as fact in the near future.

Medical research during the approach to the twenty-first century will concentrate upon the functioning of the immune system. It is already known that adverse reaction to stress reduces the immune system's ability to prevent harmful biochemical changes. For example, if the immune system is weakened, blood cholesterol levels may rise and viral infections and skin eruptions may occur. It has also been thought for some time that stress, the immune system and cancer are interlinked. Astonishing improvements have been reported by the sufferers of migraine headaches, peptic ulcers, asthma and blood pressure among other complaints when simple mental techniques to harness 'mind power' have been used. Reputable medical centres in Britain, the USA and Canada are using altered states of consciousness to programme and strengthen the body's defences against disease. This validation will certainly alter many concepts now held regarding health, ageing and disease processes. The preventive medicine of the future is likely to be increasingly concerned with the relationship between diseases and the genes to which they are linked, and in the screening programmes being developed to isolate them.

The secret of living is keeping achievement in balance with life.
The secret of life is achieving harmony between the two.

(Anonymous)

GLOSSARY

abdomen   The portion of the body lying between the lower ribs and the groin

acute   Sharp, of sudden onset

adenomatous hyperplasia   An abnormal overgrowth of the tissue lining the uterine cavity

adenomyosis   A condition where displaced fragments of endometrial (uterine lining) tissue (q.v.) are embedded abnormally in the muscular wall of the uterus (q.v.)

adrenal gland   Endocrine gland (q.v.) situated on the top of each kidney

alveoli   Group of milk-secreting cells in the breast tissue

amenorrhoea   Prolonged absence of menstruation (q.v.)

androgen   Any hormone that has a masculinising effect upon either sex

androstenedione   A chemical produced by the adrenal glands which is converted into weak oestrogen (q.v.) after a chemical change

anovulation   An absence of ovulation (q.v.)

anovulatory cycle   Menstrual cycle in which ovulation does not occur

antibody   A protein found in the blood, body fluids and tissue that binds itself to invading organisms, neutralising their effect. Antibodies are formed when antigens (q.v.) are introduced into the body

anti-cancer drugs   Chemical substances which have the power to destroy or prevent growth of cancerous or malignant cells

antigen   A foreign substance which when introduced into the body stimulates the production of antibodies

anti-prostaglandins   Drugs which prevent the formation of prosta-glandins (q.v.) by the body; may be used to relieve menstrual cramps

arteriosclerosis   Thickening of the walls of the arteries

aspiration   The removal of air, fluid or other material from a body cavity by suction (*see also* needle aspiration)

atresia   Disappearance of follicles (q.v.) within the ovary. If this happens around puberty Turner's syndrome (q.v.) may result

atrophy   Reduction in size, or wasting away

bacteria, bacterium   Microscopic organism(s) which, when abnormally present, may cause disease or infection

benign   Non-cancerous condition

biopsy   The surgical removal of tissue for the purpose of diagnosis

bone scan   A diagnostic technique, using nuclear tracer elements injected into a vein, for detecting abnormal changes in body tissue

cancer   An abnormal reproduction of cells in the body which creates one or many malignant tumours

Candida albicans   A fungus (q.v.) responsible for vaginal infection

carcinoma   A cancer. A carcinoma in situ is an early and localised cancer

cardiovascular system   The heart and blood vessels

cervical canal   Channel within the cervix (q.v.) connecting the vagina (q.v.) to the uterine cavity

cervical dysplasia   Abnormal changes of the surface cervical cells, usually benign. If severe can indicate a pre-cancerous state

cervical erosion   The replacement of normal cervical tissue on the surface of the cervix by tissue from the cervical canal. Columnar cells line the canal and have a red granular appearance. The term 'erosion' is often incorrectly applied to any redness or irritation of the cervix

cervical os   The opening leading into the cervical canal from the vagina

cervix   The lower part of the uterus, which projects into the upper part of the vagina

cholesterol   One of the fatty substances normally found in the blood. It is attached in the bloodstream to a protein which allows it to be transported via the blood vessels. It is essential for certain vital bodily processes, as well as being needed in the manufacture of hormones

chromosome   A threadlike, microscopic particle containing genetic material within the nucleus of cells

climacteric   The menopausal years

collagen   A protein in the white fibres of connective tissue (q.v.)

colporrhaphy   An operation to strengthen the pelvic floor in cases of prolapse (q.v.) of the uterus and to improve bladder control

colposcope   A binocular instrument used to magnify the surface cells of the cervix

conjugated oestrogens Oestrogens which are joined with other chemicals to improve their stability

connective tissue Sheets of fibrous tissue which support muscles and connect them to other body parts. It is composed of collagen (q.v.) and glycosaminoglycans (GAGS) (q.v.)

contraceptive A drug, device or method used to prevent pregnancy

coronary occlusion The closing or blockage of a coronary artery of the heart which may lead to a heart attack (q.v.)

corpus luteum Yellowy-pink ovarian tissue, formed after the rupture of the ovarian follicle (q.v.) and the release of its contained ovum (q.v.)

cryosurgery The use of extreme cold to destroy abnormal cells or tissue

culture A quantity of micro-organisms grown to identify the causative agent or bacteria responsible for a particular infection or disease

curettage A procedure involving the scraping of any body cavity (*see also* dilatation and curettage)

cyst A sac-like structure which may contain fluid or semi-solid material

cystitis An inflammation of the lining of the bladder, which often causes pain

cystocele A prolapse (q.v.), or bulging downwards, of the front wall of the vagina, which also displaces the bladder

diagnosis Process whereby the cause of a specific infection, disease or other condition is determined

dilatation The enlargement of any passageway

dilatation and curettage (D&C) A surgical procedure in which the cervix (q.v.) is expanded and tissue from the uterine cavity is scraped off with a curette

discharge Any abnormal or unusual secretion

disease Any abnormal or pathological condition which alters the normal functioning of the body or the mind

DNA Deoxyribonucleic acid. It is composed of two interwound chains of three substances (nucleotides): a sugar, a phosphate and a nitrogen base. The order of the base determines the genetic code. DNA is the carrier of genetic information. Each of the 46 chromosomes (q.v.) in human body cells consists of two strands of DNA containing up to 100,000 nucleotides. Along the length of each strand an average of 1,500 bases form a gene (q.v.)

dysmenorrhoea Painful menstruation

dyspareunia Painful intercourse

elastin Yellow fibres of connective tissue (q.v.)

endocervical Within the cervical canal (q.v.)

endocervical glands   Mucus-producing glands within the cervical canal

endocrine gland   One which secretes hormones directly into the bloodstream; for example, ovarian, thyroid, pituitary and adrenal glands

endometrial hyperplasia   Overgrowth of the tissue lining the uterine cavity. May be caused by uninterrupted long-term oestrogen use

endometriosis   A pelvic condition in which fragments of endometrial tissue are found outside the uterine cavity. The ovaries, back wall of the uterus and areas between the uterus and rectum are common sites

endometrium   Mucous membrane lining of the uterine cavity

equilin and **equilenin**   Oestrogens derived from the urine of pregnant mares

essential   When applied to fatty acids it refers to those that are supplied in the diet and are *essential* for life. The body is unable to manufacture them

Fallopian tubes   Two small hollow tubes, named after the Italian anatomist Gabriele Fallopius, that branch from either side of the upper part of the uterus and connect with the uterine cavity. This is the passageway in which the egg (ovum) and the sperm meet

fertilisation   The fusion of a sperm with an egg

fibroadenoma   A common benign (q.v.) breast tumour

fibrocystic breast disease   A benign breast condition in which multiple small cysts (q.v.) and fibrous tissue intertwine within normal breast tissue

fibroids   Benign tumours usually occurring in the wall of the uterus. Also known as leiomyomas (q.v.), myomas (q.v.) or fibromyomas

fimbriae   The finger-like projections at the free end of each Fallopian tube (q.v.) which guide the released egg from the ovary (q.v.) into the open end of the Fallopian tube

follicle   Ovarian sac containing an egg

follicle-stimulating hormone (FSH)   A pituitary (q.v.) hormone that causes the growth and development of ovarian follicles (q.v.)

fungus   A disease-producing organism

GAGS   An irregular, shapeless substance called glycosaminoglycans which is present between the collagen (q.v.) bundles in skin and bone. GAGS resists compression while collagen resists stretching forces. Both go to make up connective tissue (q.v.)

gene   A linear segment of DNA (q.v.) forming part of a chromosome (q.v.). Genes are the basic units of heredity

genetic code   The relationship between the nucleotide (*see* DNA) sequence in chromosomes (q.v.) and the proteins which the body manufactures, determining inherited human characteristics

genital herpes   A viral infection spread by sexual contact and caused by the herpes simplex virus. Lesions develop on and around the genitalia

genital warts Lesions on the genitalia caused by the papillomavirus; often sexually transmitted

gonadotrophin A pituitary hormone directly affecting and stimulating the gonads (q.v.). Examples are follicle-stimulating hormone (q.v.) and luteinising hormone (q.v.)

gonads Female ovaries or male testes

gynaecologist A specialist medical doctor who treats and manages problems affecting the female reproductive system

haemorrhage Abnormal heavy bleeding, either internal or external

heart attack Severe instance of heart malfunction caused by interruption of the blood circulation in the coronary arteries (a myocardial infarction)

herpes viruses A group of viruses responsible for various acute infectious conditions such as cold sores, shingles and blisters. May be responsible for some human cancers

hirsutism Excessive facial or body hair

hormonal implant A small pellet containing a hormone, such as oestrogen (q.v.) or progesterone (q.v.), which is inserted into the fat of the thigh or abdomen

hormone A complex chemical substance, produced by an endocrine gland (q.v.), which affects organs or body parts

hormone replacement therapy (HRT) The use of hormones to treat symptoms of the menopause caused by functional failure of the ovaries

hot flush/flash Sudden flow of heat to the skin, usually the upper portion of the body, accompanied by perspiration

hyperplasia An increase of cells (usually benign). In the endometrium (q.v.) this may give rise to overactivity and lead to endometrial cancer

hypothalamus The part of the brain just above the pituitary gland (q.v.) which plays a major rôle in controlling basic functions, such as appetite, sleep and body temperature

hysterectomy Surgical removal of the uterus (q.v.) and usually the cervix (q.v.), carried out either by abdominal incision or through the vagina (q.v.)

immunology The study of the body's defence mechanism (immunity) against various diseases

incontinence Lack of urinary control

infection The invasion of any tissue by harmful bacteria or organisms

infertility The temporary or permanent inability to reproduce

inflammation The reaction of tissue to infection, irritation or injury. The affected area may become painful, swollen, red and hot

insomnia   Inability to sleep

intra–uterine   Within the uterine cavity

intra–uterine contraceptive device (IUCD)   A device placed within the uterine cavity to prevent pregnancy. Examples include the coil, the loop and the shield

intra–uterine device   A device placed within the uterine cavity which releases progestogen (q.v.) to protect against endometrial cancer

in–vitro fertilisation   Fertilisation of a human egg outside the body in an artificial environment: for example, a test–tube

irradiation   The use of X–rays, radium, cobalt or other radioactive substance for diagnosis or treatment

Kegel exercises   A group of exercises for strengthening the pubo-coccygeus muscle (q.v.). Often used to improve urge incontinence

laparoscopy   A minor surgical procedure requiring an anaesthetic. An instrument with an attached light allows a surgeon to view an internal structure or organ

leiomyoma   Fibroid (q.v.) tumour of the uterus

lesion   Any unusual or abnormal tissue change; for example, a sore, growth, tumour or wart

luteinising hormone (LH)   A pituitary gonadotrophin (q.v.) which stimulates the corpus luteum (q.v.) in the ovary (q.v.) to produce progesterone (q.v.)

macrophage   Large white blood cell which has a scavenging function. It protects the body against harmful bacteria and other foreign invaders

malignant   Cancerous

mammography   An X–ray of the breast (mammary gland) using a special low–irradiation technique to detect abnormal tissue change

mastectomy   Surgical removal of a breast

masturbation   Self-stimulation to produce sexual arousal

menarche   The point at which menstruation (q.v.) begins

menopause   The point at which the last menstrual period occurs

menorrhagia   Excessively heavy bleeding during menstruation

menses   Menstrual flow

menstrual cycle   The time interval from the beginning of one menstrual period to the beginning of the next

menstruation   Monthly bleeding from the uterine cavity caused by specific hormone (q.v.) changes

mini pill   Oral contraceptive pill (q.v.) containing a small dose of progestogen (q.v.)

monilia The fungus Candida albicans (q.v.)

mucous membrane Soft, moist tissue that lines body cavities and passageways

mucus Clear secretion from a mucous membrane

myocardial infarction *See* heart attack

myoma Fibroid (q.v.) tumour of the uterus

myomectomy Surgical removal of a fibroid tumour without removal of the uterus.

needle aspiration The removal of fluid or other liquid material from a cyst (q.v.) or body cavity by means of a needle and syringe

needle biopsy The removal of a small segment of tissue by means of a special large-bore needle

nodule A lump or mass which may be either benign (q.v.) or malignant (q.v.)

oestrogen/estrogen Principal hormone produced by the ovaries (q.v.), and responsible for female sexual characteristics

Omega-3 fatty acids Essential fatty acids found in some plants and especially in oily fish; for example, linolenic acid

Omega-6 fatty acids Essential fatty acids found in plants and especially in some vegetable oils; for example, linoleic acid

oöphorectomy Surgical removal of an ovary (q.v.)

oral contraceptives Birth-control pills taken by mouth

orgasm The climax or culmination of sexual arousal, achieved by intercourse, masturbation or other sexual activity

osteoblast cells Cells associated with the formation of bone

osteoclast cells Giant cells associated with bone absorption

osteoporosis Brittleness and weakness of bones due to loss of calcium and collagen (q.v.)

ovarian resection Removal of a portion of an ovary

ovary The female sex gland or gonad (q.v.)

ovulation The discharge of an egg from the ovary

ovulatory cycle A menstrual cycle in which ovulation occurs

ovum Egg. The female sexual cell produced by the ovaries

palpate To examine an area of the body by means of touch and pressure

PAP smear A microscopic examination of cells shed from or collected from body surfaces to determine abnormal change; used routinely to screen for cancer of the cervix. The procedure is named after Dr George Papanicolaou, who invented the method

pathology The study of abnormal tissue and disease states

pelvic inflammatory disease (PID)   Any inflammation and/or infection involving the internal female genital organs

peri-menopausal   Around the time of the menopause

pituitary gland   An important endocrine gland (q.v.) located at the base of the brain

platelets   Blood cells required for normal blood clotting

polycystic ovarian syndrome   Formation of multiple small cysts on both ovaries. Signs of its presence include lack of ovulation (q.v.), infertility (q.v.), menstrual irregularities, enlarged ovaries and hirsutism (q.v.)

polyp   A mucous membrane growth, usually benign, that originates from a stalk; for example, cervical polyp, endometrial polyp, rectal polyp

premenstrual syndrome (PMS)   A collection of physical and psychological symptoms, such as tension, irritability, fatigue and abdominal bloating, that are experienced by some women a few days before menstruation commences and possibly extending into the first few days of the menstrual bleed

progesterone   The ovarian hormone produced by the corpus luteum (q.v.) following ovulation (q.v.)

progestogen   A synthetic progesterone-like hormone

prognosis   Forecast or prediction

prolactin   A pituitary gland (q.v.) hormone. High levels of this hormone may cause depression, and milk production by the mammary glands

prolapse   The downward movement of an organ, such as the uterus (q.v.), from its normal position due to poor or inadequate muscular and fibrous tissue support. *See also* cystocele, rectocele and urethrocele

proliferative endometrium   The type of endometrial tissue found during the first half of the menstrual cycle

prostaglandins   Hormone-like substances which have profound effects on various parts of the body

puberty   The age at which the sexual organs become functional

pubo-coccygeus muscle   A broad band of muscle stretching from the pubic bone to the coccyx or tail bone. The muscle helps to support the female pelvic organs and maintain their proper position

radionuclear imaging   A diagnostic technique whereby malignant (q.v.) cells are tagged with radioactive material for identification purposes (*see* bone scan)

rectocele   The prolapse, or bulging, of the rectal wall into the vagina (q.v.)

salpingitis   An infection or inflammation of the Fallopian tubes (q.v.)

salpingo-oöphorectomy   Surgical removal of a Fallopian tube and ovary

secretory endometrium The normal endometrial tissue lining the uterine cavity following ovulation (q.v.). It is produced by both oestrogen (q.v.) and progesterone (q.v.) stimulation

serum The liquid portion of blood

sign In medical terms, an abnormality detected by the examining doctor (*cf* symptom)

smear test A diagnostic procedure whereby skin cells are tested for abnormal change (*see also* PAP smear)

speculum A medical instrument which opens passageways to allow for inspection

sperm The male seed produced by the testicles

sterilisation A surgical procedure which renders men and women incapable of producing children

sterility Inability to conceive

symptom An abnormality detected by the patient (*cf* sign)

syndrome A collection of signs (q.v.) and symptoms (q.v.) which, when grouped together, constitute a medical condition

synthetic drug Man-made compound as opposed to a naturally occurring one

systemic Involving the whole body, not localised

testosterone The male sex hormone, which is also found in small amounts in women

tranquilliser A drug that has a calming sedative effect

Trichomonas vaginalis (TV) A protozoa organism which may cause infection of the vagina

Turner's syndrome A genetic defect of ovarian development due to lack of the 'Y' chromosome. Other signs are webbing of the neck, stunted growth and an absence of sexual characteristics

ultrasonography A non-invasive diagnostic technique which employs sound waves to create an image on a video screen for interpretation by a radiologist

urethra The passage leading from the bladder to the outside of the body

urethrocele A prolapse or bulging (q.v.) of the urethra into the vagina

urinalysis A common laboratory examination of the urine including microscopic review for the presence of cells, bacteria, crystals and chemical compounds

uterus The womb. The muscular organ, the size and shape of a pear, which houses the developing foetus

vaccine   Any substance which, when injected into the body, will immunise the recipient against a specific disease or infection

vagina   The birth canal extending from the uterus (q.v.) to the outside

vaginal hysterectomy   A surgical procedure in which the uterus is removed through the vagina (q.v.), often performed in conjunction with a cystocele (q.v.) or rectocele (q.v.) repair

vaginitis   An infection (q.v.) or an inflammation (q.v.) of the vagina (q.v.)

venereal warts   *See* genital warts

virus   A microscopic organism capable of producing infection, disease or other pathological condition

vulva   The female external genitalia

vulvitis   Inflammation of the vulva

womb *See* uterus

yeast   Fungus-like organism; for example, Candida albicans (q.v.)

USEFUL ADDRESSES

The following list of addresses and telephone numbers is not exhaustive: local telephone directories should yield further addresses. A woman's first point of contact should always be her own doctor, who may well refer her to a clinic not on this list.

Menopause clinics
London – NHS

Guy's Hospital
St Thomas Street, London SE1 9RT
0171-955 5000

Queen Charlotte's Hospital
399 Goldhawk Road, London
W6 0XG
0181-748 4666

Royal Free Hospital
Pond Street, London NW3 2QG
0171-794 0500

St George's Hospital
Blackshaw Road, Tooting, London
SW17 0QT
0181-672 1255

King's College Hospital
Denmark Hill, London SE5 9RS
0171-737 4000

St Thomas's Hospital
Lambeth Palace Road, London
SE1 7EH
0171-928 9292

Dulwich Hospital
East Dulwich Grove, London
SE22 8PT
0171-346 6901

Queen Mary's Hospital
Roehampton Lane, Roehampton,
London SW15 5PN
0181-789 6611

London – private

Well Woman Clinic
80 Lambeth Road, London SE1 7PW
0171-928 5633

886 Garratt Lane
London SW17 0NB
0181-672 1948

BUPA Medical Centre
(Well Woman Screening and
Menopause Clinic)
Battle Bridge House, 300 Gray's Inn
Road, London WC1X 8DU
0171-837 6484

The Amarant Trust
80 Lambeth Road, London SE1 7PW
0171-401 3855

The Marie Stopes Clinic
Marie Stopes House, 108 Whitfield
Street, London W1P 5RU
0171-388 0662

The Menopause Clinic
The Portland Hospital for
Women and Children,
205-209 Great Portland Street,
London W1N 6AH
0171-580 4400

England – NHS

Birmingham Maternity Hospital Academic Department
Queen Elizabeth Medical Centre, Edgbaston, Birmingham B15 2TG
0121-472 1377

Birmingham and Midland Hospital for Women
Showell Green Lane, Sparkhill, Birmingham B11 4HL
0121-772 1101

Woman's Hospital Gynaecological Clinic
Catherine Street, Liverpool L8 7NJ
0151-709 1000

Dryburn Hospital
North Road, Durham DH1 5TW
0191-386 4911

Newcastle General Hospital
Westgate Road, Newcastle upon Tyne NE4 6BE
0191-273 8811

George Eliot Hospital
College Street, Nuneaton, Warwickshire CV10 7DJ
NUNEATON (01203) 351351

Beckenham Hospital
379 Croydon Road, Beckenham, Kent BR3 3QL
0181-289 6600

Nottingham City Hospital
Hucknall Road, Nottingham NG5 1PB
NOTTINGHAM (0115) 9691169

Hull Royal Infirmary
Anlaby Road, Kingston upon Hull HU3 2JX
KINGSTON UPON HULL (01482) 328541

Northern General Hospital
Gynaecology Department, Herries Road, Sheffield S5 7AU
SHEFFIELD (0114) 2434343

Royal Liverpool Hospital
Prescot Street, Liverpool L7 8XP
0151-706 2000

The Menopause Clinic
Department of Obstetrics and Gynaecology, The Royal Oldham Hospital, Rochdale Road, Oldham, Lancashire OL1 2JH
0161-624 0420

Hospital of St Cross
Barby Road, Rugby, Warwickshire CV22 5PX
RUGBY (01788) 572831

Stafford District General Hospital
Weston Road, Stafford ST16 3SA
STAFFORD (01785) 57731

England – private

32 Westbourne Villas
Hove, East Sussex BN3 1GF
BRIGHTON (01273) 720217

Haslemere House
68 Haslemere Avenue, Mitcham, Surrey CR4 3BA
0181-648 3234

31 Rodney Street
Liverpool L1 9EH
0151-709 8522

25 Britannia Pavilion
Albert Dock, Liverpool L3 4AA
0151-709 3998

Others – formerly FPA clinics

Central Health Clinic
1 Mulberry Street, Sheffield S1 2PJ
SHEFFIELD (0114) 2716790

Fairfields Clinic
5 Quers Street, Basingstoke, Hampshire RG21 1PT
BASINGSTOKE (01256) 26980

Greenhouse
Trevelyan Terrace, Bangor, Gwynedd LL57 1AX
BANGOR (01248) 352176

British Pregnancy Advisory Services
160 Shepherd's Bush Road, London W6 7PB
0171-602 2723

Central Clinic
Victoria House, Park Street, Kingston
upon Hull HU2 8TD
KINGSTON UPON HULL (0148) 2223191

Scotland – NHS

Glasgow Royal Infirmary
Castle Street, Glasgow G4 0SF
0141-552 3535

Stobhill Hospital
133 Balornock Road, Glasgow
G21 3UW
0141-558 0111

Glasgow Western Infirmary
Dunbarton Road, Glasgow G11 6NT
0141-211 2000

Family Planning Clinic
18 Dean Terrace, Edinburgh EH4 1NL
0131-332 7941

Northern Ireland

Royal Victoria Hospital
Grosvenor Road, Belfast BT12 6BA
(01232) 240503

Republic of Ireland – general

For Dublin, Republic of Ireland, the
prefix is 00 3531

Coombe Women's Hospital
Dolphin's Barn Street, Dublin 8
DUBLIN 4537561

Irish Family Planning Information Office
Halfpenny Court, 37 Lower Ormand
Quay, Dublin 1
DUBLIN 872 5033

Irish Family Planning Association
Cathal Brugha Street Clinic,
Dublin 1
DUBLIN 8727276

Irish Family Planning Association
69 Synge Street, Dublin 8
DUBLIN 6682420

Rotunda Hospital
Parnell Square West, Dublin 1
DUBLIN 8730700

Well Woman Clinic
35 Lower Liffey Street, Dublin 1
DUBLIN 6728051

Family Planning Services
67 Pembroke Road, Dublin 4
DUBLIN 6683714

Counselling and information

The Amarant Trust
80 Lambeth Road, London SE1 7PW
0171-401 3855

BACUP (British Association of Cancer United Patients)
0800-181199
Professional advice.

CancerLink
0171-833 2451/0131-228 5557

Cancer Relief Macmillan Fund
15-19 Britten Street, London SW3 3TZ
0171-351 7811
Funds breast-care nurses

Cancer Research Campaign
0171-224 1333

The Marie Stopes Clinic
Marie Stopes House, 108 Whitfield
Street, London W1P 5RU
0171-388 0662

Marriage Guidance London
76a New Cavendish Street, London
W1M 7LB
0171-580 1087

National Health Information Service
0800-665544

Relate (National Marriage Guidance Council)
Herbert Gray College, Little Church
Street, Rugby, Warwickshire
CV21 3AP
RUGBY (01788) 573241

UPCS (see page 134)
0800-387326 for further information on
this contraceptive system.

Well Woman Clinic
Palatine Centre, 63-65 Palatine Road,
Withington, Manchester M20 9LJ
0161-434 3555

Well Woman Clinic
Wythenshaw Health Care Centre,
Stancliffe Road, Sharston, Manchester
M22 4PJ
0161-946 0065

Women's Health Concern
(please enclose sae)
PO Box 1629
London W8 6AU
0181-556 1966

**Women's Nationwide Cancer Control
Campaign**
0171-729 4688
Screening information.

For information on **clinical trials of
new HRT treatments in the London
area:** 0171-486 7641

Pregnancy

**British Pregnancy Advisory Service
(BPAS)**
7 Belgrave Road, London SW1V 1QB
0171-828 2484
For other branches in England, Scotland
and Wales, call (01564) 793225

Support groups

**Breast Care and Mastectomy Association
of Great Britain**
15-19 Britten Street, London SW3 3TZ
0171-867 1103

Carers National Association
20-25 Glasshouse Yard, London
EC1A 4JS
0171-490 8898

Central Council of Physical Recreation
Francis House, Francis Street, London
SW1P 1DE
0171-828 3163

Cruse – Bereavement Care
Cruse House, 126 Sheen Road,
Richmond, Surrey TW9 1UR
0181-940 4818

Family Planning Association
27 Mortimer Street, London
W1N 7RJ
0171-636 7866

Lymphoedema Support Group
0171-727 6973

British Migraine Association
178a High Road, West Byfleet, Surrey
KT14 7ED
WEYBRIDGE (01932) 352468

National Osteoporosis Society
PO Box 10, Radstock, Bath BA3 3YB
RADSTOCK (01761) 432472

The Institute of Psychosexual Medicine
Cavendish Square, 11 Chandos Street,
London W1M 9DE
0171-580 0631

**SPOD (Association to Aid the Sexual
and Personal Relationships of People
with Disabilities)**
286 Camden Road, London N7 0BJ
0171-607 8851

Tenovus Cancer Information Centre
11 Whitchurch Road, Cardiff
CF4 3JN
CARDIFF (01222) 621543

National Association of Widows
54-57 Alison Street, Digbeth,
Birmingham B5 5TH
0121-643 8348

**Women's Health and Reproductive
Rights Information Centre**
52-54 Featherstone Street, London
EC1Y 8RT
0171-251 6580

**Women's Nationwide Cancer Control
Campaign**
Suna House, 128-130 Curtain Road,
London EC2A 3AR
0171-729 4688

National Women's Register
9 Bank Plain, Norwich, Norfolk
NR2 4SL
NORWICH (01603) 406767

Complementary representative bodies

Acupuncture
British Medical Acupuncture Society,
Newton House, Newton Lane,
Whitley, Warrington,
Cheshire WA4 4JA
WARRINGTON (01925) 730727

Alexander Technique
The Society of Teachers of the
Alexander Technique (STAT),
20 London House, 266 Fulham Road,
London SW10 9EL
0171-351 0828

Aromatherapy
International Federation of
Aromatherapists, 4 Eastmearn Road,
West Dulwich, London SE21 8HA
0181-742 2605

Reflexology
The British School of Reflexology,
92 Sheering Road, Old Harlow, Essex
CM17 0JW
HARLOW (01279) 429060

Shiatsu
Shiatsu Society, 5 Foxcote,
Wokingham, Berkshire RG11 3PG
WOKINGHAM (01734) 730836

Stress
Centre for Autogenic Training, Positive
Health Centre, 100 Harley Street,
London W1N 1DF
0171-935 1811

Yoga
The British Wheel of Yoga, 1 Hamilton
Place, Boston Road, Sleaford,
Lincolnshire NG34 7ES
SLEAFORD (01529) 306851

BIBLIOGRAPHY

Chapter 1 The menstrual cycle

Gosden, R.G. 1985. *Biology of Menopause: the causes and consequences of ovarian ageing.* London, Academic Press

Siiteri, P.K. & MacDonald P.C. 1973. The role of extraglandular estrogen in human endocrinology. In *Handbook of Physiology,* eds. R.O. Greep & E.B. Ashwood, section 7, Endocrinology vol II, part I, pp. 615-29. Washington, American Physiological Society

Vermulen, A. 1976. The hormonal activity of the post-menopausal ovary. *J Clin Endocrinol Metab,* **42,** 247-53

Sherman, B.M. & Wallace, R.B. 1985. Menstrual patterns: menarche through menopause. In *Mechanism of Menstrual Bleeding,* eds. D.T. Baird & E.A. Michie, vol 25, pp. 157-63. New York, Raven Press

Wide, L. 1989. Follicle-stimulating hormones in anterior pituitary glands from children and adults differ in relation to sex and age. *J Endocrinol,* **123,** 519-29

Van Look, P.F.A., Lothian, H., Hunter, W.M., Michie, E.A., Baird, D.T. 1977. Hypothalmic-pituitary-ovarian function in peri-menopausal women. *Clin Endocrinol,* **7,** 13-31

Tataryn, I.V., Meldrum, D.R., Lu, J.K.H., Frumar, A.M., Judd, H.L. 1979. LH, FSH and skin temperature during the menopausal hot flush. *J Clin Endocrinol Metab,* **49,** 152-4

Gambone, J., Meldrum, D.R., Laufer, L., Chang, R.J., Lu, J.K.H., Judd, H.L. 1984. Further delineation of hypothalmic dysfunction responsible for menopausal hot flushes. *J Clin Endocrinol Metab,* **59,** 1097-102

Baker, T.G. 1971. Radiosensitivity of mammalian oocytes with particular reference to the human female. *Am J Obstet Gynecol,* **110,** 746-61

de Jong, F.H. & Sharpe, R.M. 1976. Evidence for inhibin-like activity in bovine follicular fluid. *Nature,* **263,** 71-2

Bäckstrom, C.T., Boyle, H., Baird, D.T. 1981. Persistence of symptoms of premenstrual tension in hysterectomised women. *Brit J Obstet Gynaecol,* **88,** 530-6

Dalton, K. 1984. *The Premenstrual Syndrome and Progesterone Therapy.* 2nd ed. Chicago, Year Book Medical Publishers

McKinlay, S., Jeffreys, M., Thompson, B. 1972. An investigation of the age at menopause. *J Biosocial Science,* **4,** 161-73

Treloar, A. 1982. Predicting the close of menstrual life. In *Changing Perspectives on Menopause*, eds. A.M. Voda, M. Dinnerstein, S. O'Donnell. Austin, Univ of Texas Press

Wilson, R.C.D. 1989. PMS. Timing of symptoms is key to diagnosis. *Modern Medicine*, **34,** 921-6

Wilson, R.C.D. 1990. PMS. Treatment update. *Modern Medicine*, **35,** 24-30

Baker, T.G. 1972. Oögenesis and ovulation. In *Reproduction in mammals. I: Germ cells and fertilization*, eds. C.R. Austin, R.V. Short, Cambridge University Press, Cambridge, 14-45

Faddy, M.J., Gosden, R.G., Gougeon, A., Richardson, S.J., Nelson, J.F. 1992. Accelerated disappearance of ovarian follicles in mid-life: implications for forecasting menopause. *Human Reprod*, **7,** 1342-6

Nock, B. 1986. Nor-andrengenic regulation of Progestin Receptors: New findings, new questions. In *Reproduction: A Behavioural and Neuroendocrine Prospective*, eds. B.R. Komusaruk *et al*, New York: *Am J N Y Acad Sci*, 415-22

Nakajima, S.T., Gibson, M. 1989. The effect of a meal on circulating steady-state progesterone. 1989. *J Clin Endo Met*, **69,** 917-19

Yen, S.S.C., Jaffe, R.B. 1991 *Reproductive Endocrinology*. London: W.B. Saunders

Rannevik, G. 1986. A prospective long-term study in women from premonopause to postmenopause: Changing profiles of gonadotrophins, oestrogens and androgens. *Maturitas*, **8,** 297-307

Chapter 2 Symptoms and signs of the menopause

Voda, A.M. 1981. Climacteric hot flash. *Maturitas*, **3,** 73-90

Sturdee, D.W., Wilson, K.A., Pipili, E., Crocker, A.D. 1978. Physiological aspects of the menopausal hot flush. *Br Med J*, **ii,** 79-80

Bungay, G.T., Vessey, M.P., McPherson, K. 1980. Study of symptoms in middle life with special reference to the menopause. *Br Med J*, **ii,** 55-64

Dennerstein, L. & Burrows, G.D. 1978. A review of the studies of the psychological symptoms found at the menopause. *Maturitas*, **1,** 55-64

Masters, W.H. & Johnson, V.E. 1966. *Human Sexual Response*. Boston, Little Brown

Leiblum, Sr., Bachmann, G.A., Kemmann, E. *et al.* 1983. Vaginal atrophy in the post-menopausal woman. *J Am Med Assoc*, **249,** 2195-8

Hammarback, S., Bäckstrom, T., Holst, J. *et al.* 1985. Cyclical mood changes as in the premenstrual syndrome during sequential estrogen-progestogen post-menopausal replacement therapy. *Acta Obstet Gynecol Scand*, **64,** 393-7

Van Keep, P.A. & Kellerhals, J.M. 1974. The impact of socio-cultural factors on symptom formation. *Psychother Psychosom*, **23,** 251-63

Glenn, N.D. 1975. Psychological well-being in the post-parental stage: some evidence from national surveys. *J Marriage Fam*, **37,** 105-10

Collins, A., Hanson, U., Eneroth, P. 1983. Post-menopausal symptoms and response to hormonal replacement therapy: influence of psychological factors. *J Psychosom Obstet Gynaecol*, **2,** 227-33

Sarrel, P.M. & Whitehead, M.I. 1985. Sex and menopause: defining the issues. *Maturitas*, **7,** 217-24

Versi, E., Brincat, M., Cardozo, L.D., O'Dowd, T., Cooper, D., Studd, J.W.W. 1988. Correlation of urethral physiology and skin collagen in post-menopausal women. *Br J Obstet Gynaecol*, **2,** 147-52

Savvas, M., Treasure, J., Studd, J.W.W., Fogelman, I., Moniz, C., Brincat, M. 1989. The effect of anorexia nervosa on skin thickness, skin collagen and bone density. *Br J Obstet Gynaecol*, **96**, 1392-4

Watson, N.R., Studd, J.W.W., Riddle, A.F., Savvas, M. 1988. Suppression of ovulation by transdermal oestradiol patches. *Br Med J*, **297**, 900-1

Jaszmann, L. 1973. Epidemiology of climacteric and post-climacteric complaints. In *Ageing and Oestrogens*, eds. P.A. Van Keep & C. Lauritzen, pp. 22-5. Basel, Karger

Magos, A.L., Brincat, M., Studd, J.W.W. 1986. Treatment of the premenstrual syndrome by subcutaneous oestradiol implants and cyclical oral norethisterone – a placebo controlled study. *Br Med J*, **1**, 1629-33

Gelder, M.G., Gath, D., Mayou, R. 1989. *Oxford Textbook of Psychiatry*, 2nd ed. London, OUP

American Psychiatric Association. 1987. *Diagnostic and Statistical Manual of Mental Disorders*, 3rd ed. revd. Washington DC, American Psychiatric Association

Hamilton, M. 1967. Development of a rating scale for primary depressive illness. *Br J Soc Clin Psychol*, **6**, 278-96

Iatrakis, G., Haronis, N., Sakellaropoulos, G., Kourkabas, A., Gallos, M. 1986. Psychosomatic symptoms of post-menopausal women with or without hormonal treatment. *Psychother Psychosom*, **46**, 116-21

Brecher, E.M. 1983. *Love, Sex and Ageing*. Consumers Union Report, Little Brown

Stevenson, R.W.D., Szasz, G., Lee, L.M. 1988. Erection dysfunction: therapy options. *Brit Col Med J*, **30**, 95-7

Rinehart, J.S. & Schiff, I. 1985. Sexuality and the menopause. In *Human Sexuality: psychosexual effects of disease*, M. Farber. NY, Macmillan

Improving Government Statistics: gaps and discontinuities in official statistics. Monitoring hospital in-patient enquiry data, Social Science Forum, September 1991

Kaufert, P.A., Gilbert, P., Hassard, T. 1988. Researching the symptoms of menopause: An exercise in methodology. *Maturitas*, **10**, 117-31

McKinlay, S.M., Brambilla, P.J., Posner, J.G. 1992. The normal menopause transition. *Maturitas*, **14**, 103-15

McKinley, S., Jeffreys, M. 1974. The menopausal syndrome. *Br J Prev Soc Med*, **28**, 108-15

Neugarten, B.L., Kraines, R.J. 1965. Menopausal symptoms in women of various ages. *Psychosom Med*, **27**, 266-73

Thompson, B., Hart, S.A., Durno, D. 1973. Menopausal age and symptomatology in general practice. *J Biol Sci*, **5**, 71

Lu, J.K.H., Judd, H.L. 1991. The neuroendocrine aspects of menopausal hot flushes. In The Climacteric Hot Flush, ed. E. Schonbaum, *Prog Basic Clin Pharmacol*. Basel: Karger, **6**, 83-99

Dennerstein, L. 1987. Depression in the menopause. *Obstet Gynecol Clin North Am*, **4**, 33-48

Depression, inflammatory disease linked to oestrogen. *J Clin Invest* (US), October 1993

McEwen, B.S. 19988. Basic research perspective: Ovarian hormone influence on brain neurochemical function. In *Contemporary issues in obstetrics and gynecology: The premenstrual syndromes*, ed. I.H. Gise. New York: Churchill-Livingstone, 21-33

Hamilton, J. Estrogen, memory and Alzheimer's disease. 1994. *Can Med Assoc J*, Nov. **15**, 1465-7

Cullberg, G., Hamberger, L., Mattsson, L-A, Mobacken, H., Samsioe, G. 1985. Effects of a low-dose desogestrel-ethinyloestradiol combination on hirsutism, androgens and sex hormone binding globulin in women with a polycystic ovary syndrome. *Acata Obstet Gynecol Scand*, **64**(3), 195-202

Chapter 3 Osteoporosis

Albright, F., Smith, P.H., Richardson, A.M. 1941. Post-menopausal osteoporosis – its clinical features. *J Am Med Assoc*, **116**, 2465-74

Alberts, B., Bray, D., Lewis, T. *et al.* 1983. Cell-cell adhesion and the extracellular matrix. In *Molecular Biology of the Cell*, ed. B. Alberts, pp. 673-715. NY, Garland Pub

Forbes, R.M., Cooper, A.R., Mitchell, L. 1953. The composition of the adult human body as determined by chemical analysis. *J. Biol Chem*, **203**, 359-66

Birkenhager-Frenkel, D.H. 1966. Assessment of porosity in bone specimens, differences in chemical composition between normal bone and bone from patients with senile osteoporosis. In *Fourth European Symposium on Calcified Tissues*, ed. P.J. Gaillard, pp. 8-9. Amsterdam, Excerpta Medica

Hoffenberg, R., James, O.F.W., Brocklehurst, J.C. *et al.* 1989. Fractured neck of femur. Prevention and management. *J R Coll Physicians London*, **23**, 8-12

Cooper, C., Barker, D.J.P., Morris, J., Briggs, R.S. 1987. Osteoporosis falls and age in fracture of the proximal femur. *Br Med J*, **295**, 13-15

Ross, P.D., Wasnich, R.D., Vogel, J.M. 1988. Detection of pre-fracture spinal osteoporosis using bone mineral absorptiometry. *J Bone Miner Res*, **3**, 1-11

Hui, S.L., Slemenda, C.S., Johnston, C.C. 1988. Age and bone mass as predictors of fracture in a prospective study. *J Clin Invest*, **81**, 1804-9

Odvina, C.V., Wergedal, J.E., Libanati, C.R., Schulz, F.E., Baylink, D.J. 1988. Relationship between trabecular vertebral bone density and fractures: a quantitative definition of spinal osteoporosis. *Metabolism*, **37**, 221-8

Slemenda, C.S., Hui, S.L., Longscope. C. *et al.* 1987. Sex steroids and bone mass: a study of changes about the time of the menopause. *J Clin Invest*, **80**, 1261

Gordan, G.S. & Genant, H.K. 1978. Post-menopausal osteoporosis is a preventable disease. *Contemporary Obstetrics and Gynaecology*, **11**, 47

Frost, H.M. 1964. Dynamics of bone remodelling. In *Bone Biodynamics*, pp. 315. Boston, Little Brown

Stevenson, J.C. *et al.* 1989. Determinants of bone density in normal women; risk factors for future osteoporosis. *Br Med J*, **298**, 924-8

Ciccarelli, E., Savino, L., Carlevetto, V., Bertagna, A., Isaia, G.C., Cammanni, I. 1988. Vertebral bone density in non-amenorrhoeic hyperprolactinaemic women. *Clin Endocrinol*, **67**, 124-30

Rigotti, N.A., Nussbaum, S.R., Herzog, D.B., Neer, R.M. 1984. Osteoporosis in women with anorexia nervosa. *N Engl J Med*, **311**, 1601-6

Eriksen, E.F., Colvard, D.S., Berg, N.J., Graham, M.L., Mann, K.G., Spelsberg, T.C., Riggs, B.L. 1988. Evidence of estrogen receptors in normal human osteoblast cells. *Science*, **241**, 84-6

McNair, P., Christiansen, C., Christiansen, M.S. *et al.* 1981. Development of bone mineral loss in insulin-treated diabetes: a 12-year follow-up study in 60 patients. *Eur J Clin Invest*, **11**, 55-9

Prior, J.C. 1990. Progesterone as a bone-trophic hormone. *Endocrine Reviews by the Endocrine Society*, vol ii, no **2**, pp. 386-98

Central Statistical Office. 1987. *Social Trends no 17*. London, HMSO

Office of Population Censuses and Surveys. 1987. *Hospital in-patient enquiry*. London, HMSO

Holbrook, T.L., Grazier, K., Kelsey, J.L., Stauffer, R.N. 1987. *The frequency of occurrence, impact and cost of selected musculoskeletal conditions in the United States*. Chicago, Am Academy of Orthopedic Surgeons

Royal College of Physicians Report. 1989. *Fractured neck of femur – prevention and management*. London, RCP

Horsman, A., Burkinshaw, L., Pearson, D., Oxby, C.B., Milner, R.M. 1983. Estimating total body calcium from peripheral bone measurements. *Calcif Tiss Int*, **35**, 135-44

Mazess, R.B. & Wahner, H.M. 1988. Nuclear medicine and densitometry. In *Osteoporosis: etiology, diagnosis and management*, eds. B.L. Riggs & J.L. Melton III, pp. 251-95. NY, Raven Press

Sartoris, D.J. & Resnick, D. 1989. Dual-energy radiographic absorptiometry for bone densitometry: current status and perspective. *Am J Radiol*, **152**, 214-16

Leblanc, A.D., Evans, H.J., Marsh, C., Schneider, V., Johnson, P.C., Jhingran, S.G. 1986. Precision of dual-photon absorptiometry measurements. *J Nucl Med*, **27**, 1362-5

Edwards, L. 1989. New research data on hormone replacement therapy. *Symposium Newsletter*, issue **9**. Bath, Nat Osteo Soc

Hansen, M.A. 1991. Role of peak bone mass and loss in post-menopausal osteoporosis: 12-year study. *Br Med J*, **303**, 961-4

WHO. 1982. *World Health Statistics Quarterly*, **35**, 11

Castelli, W.P. 1988. Cardiovascular disease in women. *Am J Obstet Gynecol*, **95**, 1554

Gordon, T., Kannel, W.B., Hjortland, M.C., McNamara, P.M. 1978. Menopause and coronary heart disease: the Framingham study. *Ann Intern Med*, **89**, 157-61

Pettiti, D., Perlman, J., Sidney, S. 1987. Non-contraceptive oestrogens and mortality: long-term follow-up of women in the Walnut Creek study. *Obstet Gynecol*, **70**, 289-93

Henderson, B.E., Ross, R.K., Paganini-Hill, A., Mack, T.M. 1986. Estrogen use and cardiovascular disease. *Am J Obstet Gynecol*, **154**, 1181-6

Notelovitz, M., Kitchens, C.S., Ware, M.D. 1984. Coagulation and fibrinolysis in estrogen-treated surgically menopausal women. *Obstet Gynecol*, **63**, 621-4

Ross, R.K. & Paganini-Hill, A. 1983. Estrogen replacement therapy and coronary heart disease. *Sem Reprod Endocrinol*, **1**, 19-25

The Surgeon General's Report on Health Promotion and Disease Prevention. 1979. *Healthy People*. DHEW (PHS) Publication no 79-55071. Washington DC, US Govt Print Office

Bush, T.L., Barrett-Conner, E., Cowan, L.D. *et al.* 1987. *Cardiovascular mortality and non-contraceptive use of estrogen in women: results from the Lipid Research Clinics program follow-up study*, **75**, 1102-9

Meade, T.W. 1987. The epidemiology of haemostasis and other variables in coronary artery disease. In *Thrombosis and Haemostasis*, eds. M. Verstraete, J. Vermylen, R. Lijnen, J. Arnout, pp. 37-60. Leuven, Leuven Univ Press

Vickers, M.V. & Thompson, S.G. 1985. Sources of variability in dose response platelet aggregometry. *Thromb Haemost*, **53**, 216-20

Alberts, B., Bray, D., Lewis, T. *et. al.* 1983. Cell-cell adhesion and the extracellular matrix. In *Molecular biology of the cell*, ed. B. Alberts. New York: Garland Publishing, 673-715

Wolman, R.L. 1994. Osteoporosis and Exercise. *Br Med J*, **309**, 400-3

Brincat, M., Studd, J.W.W. 1988. Skin and the menopause. In *The menopause*, ed. J.W.W. Studd, M.I. Whitehall. Oxford: Blackwell Scientific Publications, 85-101

Lindsay, R. 1987. Estrogen therapy in the prevention and management of osteoporosis. *Am J Obstet Gynecol*, **156**, 1347-57

Lindsay, R., Hart, D.M., Aiken, J.M. *et al.* 1976. Long-term prevention of postmenopausal osteoporosis by oestrogen: Evidence for an increased bone mass after delayed onset of oestrogen treatment. *The Lancet,* **1,** 1038-41

Chestnut, C.H.III., Sisom, K., Nelp, W.B. *et al.* 19834. Are synthetic salmon calcitonin and anabolic steroids efficacious in the treatment of postmenopausal osteoporosis. In *Osteoporosis: a multidisciplinary problem,* ed. A. St J. Dixon *et al.* Royal Society of Medicine, *Int Congress and symposium* series, **55,** 239-44

Reid, I.R., Ames, R.W., Sharpe, S.J. *et al.* 1992. Effect of calcium supplementation on bone loss in postmenopausal women. *New Engl J Med,* **328,** 460-4

Chapter 4 Cardiovascular disease

[1] WHO. 1982. *World Health Statistics Quarterly,* **35,** 11

[2] Castelli, W.P. 1988. Cardiovascular disease in women. *Am J. Obstet Gynecol,* **95,** 1554

[3] Gordon, T., Kannel, W.B., Hjortland, M.C., McNamara, P.M. 1978. Menopause and coronary heart disease: the Framingham study. *Ann Intern Med,* **89,** 157-61

[4] Pettiti, D., Perlman, J., Sidney, S. 1987. Non-contraceptive oestrogens and mortality: long-term follow-up of women in the Walnut Creek study. *Obstet Gynecol,* **70,** 289-93

[5] Lerner, D.J., Kannel, W.B. 1986. Patterns of coronary heart disease morbidity and mortality in the sexes: a 26-year follow-up of the Framingham population. *Am Heart J,* **111,** 383-90

[6] Kannel, W.B., Feinleib, M. 1972. Natural history of angina pectoris in the Framingham study: Prognosis and survival. *Am J Cardiol,* **29,** 154-63

[7] Kannel, W.B., Abbott, R.D. 1987. Incidence and prognosis of myocardial infarction in women: The Framingham Study. In *Coronary heart disease in women,* eds. E.D. Eaker, B. Packard, N.K. Wenger, T.B. Clarkson, H.A. Tyroler. New York: Haymarket Doyma, 208-14

[8] Ayanian, J.Z., Epstein, A.M. 1991. Differences in the use of procedures between women and men hospitalised for coronary heart disease. *N Engl J Med,* **325,** 221-5

[9] Steingart, R.M., Packer, M., Hamm, P. *et al.* 1991. Sex differences in the management of coronary artery disease. *N Engl J Med,* **325,** 226-30

[10] Weiner, D.A., Ryan, T.J., McCabe, C.H. *et al.* 1979. Exercise stress testing: Correlations among history of angina, ST-segment response and prevalence of coronary-artery disease in the Coronary Artery Surgery Study (CASS). *N Engl J Med,* **301,** 230-5

[11] Robert, A.R., Melin, J.A., Detry, J-M.R. 1991. Logistic discriminant analysis improves diagnostic accuracy of exercise testing for coronary artery disease in women. *Circulation,* **83,** 1202-9

[12] Tobin, J.N., Wassertheil-Smoller, S., Wexler, J.P. *et al.* 1987. Sex bias in considering coronary bypass surgery. *Ann Intern Med,* **107,** 19-25

[13] Pedersen, T.R. 1985. Six-year follow-up of the Norwegian Multicenter Study on timolol after acute myocardial infarction. *N Engl J Med,* **313,** 1055-8

[14] ISIS-2 (Second International Study of Infarct Survival) Collaborative Group. 1988. Randomised trial of intravenous streptokinase, oral aspirin, both, or neither among 17,187 cases of suspected acute myocardial infarction: ISIS-2. *The Lancet,* **2,** 349-60

[15] Boogaard, M.A.K., Briody, M.E. 1985. Comparison of the rehabilitation of men and women post-myocardial infarction. *J Cardiopulmonary Rehabil,* **5,** 379-84

[16] Krumholtz, H.M., Douglas, P.S., Lauer, M.S., Pasternak, R.C. 1992. Selection of patients for coronary angiography and coronary revascularization early after

myocardial infarction: Is there evidence for a gender bias? *Ann Intern Med,* **116,** 785-90

[17] Sawada, S.G., Ryan, T., Fineberg, N.S., *et al.* Exercise echocardiographic detection of coronary artery disease in women. *J Am Coll Cardiol,* **14,** 1440-7

[18] Masini, M., Picano, E., Lattanzi, F., Distante, A., L'Abbate, A. 1988. High-dose dipyridamole-echocardiography test in women: Correlation with exercise-electrocardiography test and coronary arteriography. *J Am Coll Cardiol,* **12,** 682-5

[19] Grady. D., Rubin, S.M., Petitti, D.B. *et al.* 1992. Hormone therapy to prevent disease and prolong life in postmenopausal women. *Ann Intern Med,* **117,** 1016-37

[20] Henderson, B.E., Ross, R.K., Paganini-Hill, A., Mack, T.M. 1986. Estrogen use and cardiovascular disease. *Am J Obstet Gynecol,* **164,** 1181-6

[21] Notelovitz, M., Kitchens, C.S., Watre, M.D. 1984. Coagulation and fibrinolysis in estrogen-treated surgically menopausal women. *Obstet Gynecol,* **63,** 621-4

[22] Ross, R.K. & Paganini-Hill, A. 1983. Estrogen replacement therapy and coronary heart disease. *Sem Reprod Endocrinol,* **1,** 19-25

[23] Bush, T.L., Barrett-Conner, E., Cowan, L.D. *et al.* 1987. Cardiovascular mortality and non-contraceptive use of estrogen in women: results from the Lipid Research Clinics program follow-up study, **75,** 1102-9

[24] Meade, T.W. 1987. The epidemiology of haemostasis and other variables in coronary artery disease. In *Thrombosis and Haemostasis,* eds. M. Verstraete, J. Vermylen, R. Lijnen, J. Arnout, pp. 37-60. Leuven, Leuven Univ Press

[25] Jiang, C., Sarrel, P.M., Lindsay, D.C., Poole-Wilson, P.A., Collins, P. 1991. Endothelium-independent relxation of rabbit coronary artery by 17B-estradiol in vitro. *Br J Pharmacol,* **104,** 1033-7

[26] Collins, P., Rosano, G.M.E., Jiang, C., Lindsay, D., Sarrel, P.M., Poole-Wilson, P.A. 1993. Cardiovascular protection by estrogen – a calcium antagonist effect? *The Lancet,* **341,** 1264-5

[27] Rosano, G.M.C., Sarrel, P.M., Pole-Wilson, P.A., Collins, P. 1993. Effects of acute administration of oestradiol-17 on exercise-induced myocardial ischemia in female patients with coronary artery disease. *The Lancet,* **342,** 133

[28] Jiang, C., Sarrel, P.M., Poole-Wilson, P.A., Collins, P. 1991. Acute effects of 17-estradiol rabbit coronary artery contractile response to endothelin. *Am J Physiol,* **263** (Heart Circ Physiol 32), H271

[29] Grady, D., Ruben, S.M., Petitti, D.M. *et al.* 1992. Hormone therapy to prevent disease and prolong life in postmenopausal women. *Ann Int Med,* **117,** 1016-39

[30] Crook, D., Cust, M.P., Gangar, K.F. *et al.* 19921. Comparison of transdermal and oral estrogen/progestin hormone replacement therapy: effects of serum lipids and lipoproteins. *Am J Obstet Gynecol,* **166,** 950-5

[31] Gordon, D.J., Probstfield, J.L., Garrison, R.J., Neaton, J.D., Castelli, W.P., Knoke, J.D., Jacobs, D.R., Bangdiwala, S., Tyroler, H.A. 1989. High-density lipoprotein cholesterol and cardiovascular disease. Four prospective American studies. *Circularion,* **79,** 8-15

[32] Sandkamp, M., Assmann, G. 1990. Lipoprotein (a) in PROCAM participants and young myocardial infarction survivors. In *Lipoprotein (a): 25 Years of Progress,* ed. A.M. Scanu. Orlando, Fla: Academic Press Inc, 205-10

[33] Meade, T.W., Berra, A. 1992. Hormone replacement therapy and cardiovascular disease. *Br Med Bull,* **48,** 276-308

[34] Colditz, G.A., Willett, W.C., Stampfer, M.J. *et al.* 1987. Menopause and the risk of coronary heart disease. *N Engl J Med,* **316,** 1105-10

[35] Vague, J. 1956. The degree of masculine differentiation of obesities: a factor determining predisposition to diabetes, atherosclerosis, gout and uric calculus disease. *Am J Clin Nutr,* **4**, 20-34

[36] Hauner, H., Bognar, E., Blum, A. 1994. Body fat distribution and its association with metabolic and hormonal risk factors in women with angiographically assessed coronary artery disease. Evidence for the presence of a metabolic syndrome. *Atherosclerosis,* **105**, 209-16

[37] Walton, C., Godsland, I.F., Proudler, A.J., Wynn, V., Stevenson, J.C. 1993. The effects of the menopause on insulin sensitivity, secretion and elimination in non-obese, healthy women. *Eur J Clin Invest,* **23**, 466-73

[38] Reaven, G.M. 1988. Role of insulin resistance in human disease. *Diabetes,* **37**, 1595-607

[39] Godsland, I.F., Gangar, K.F., Walton, C. *et al.* 1993. Insulin resistance, secretion and elimination in postmenopausal women receiving oral or transdermal hormone replacement therapy. *Metabolism,* **42**, 846-53

Chapter 5 Managing the menopause with hormone replacement therapy

Ziel, H. & Finkle, W. 1975. Increased risk of endometrial carcinoma among users of conjugated oestrogens. *N Engl J Med,* **293**, 1167-70

Vaishnav, R., Gallagher, J.A., Beresford, J.N., Poser, J., Russell, R.G.G. 1984. Direct effects of stanozolol and oestrogens in human bone cell culture. In *Osteoporosis,* ed. C. Christiansen *et al,* pp. 485-8. Copenhagen, Gostrup Hospital

Consensus development conference. 1987. Prophylaxis and treatment of osteoporosis. *Br Med J,* **295**, 914-16

Editorial. 1987. Osteoporosis. *The Lancet,* **ii**, 833-5

Crilly, R.G., Francis, R.M., Nordin, B.E.C. 1981. Steroid hormones, ageing and bone. *J Clin Endocrinol Metab,* **10**, 115-39

Cundy, T., Evans, M. *et al.* 1991. Bone density in women receiving depot MPA for contraception. *Br Med J,* **303**, 13-16

Mashchak, C.A., Lobo, R.A., Dozono-Takano, R. *et al.* 1982. Comparison of pharmacodynamic properties of various estrogen formulations. *Am J Obstet Gynecol,* **244**, 511-18

Aylward, M., Maddock, J., Lewis, P.A. *et al.* 1977. Oestrogen replacement therapy and blood clotting. *Curr Med Res Opin,* **4**, (suppl 3), 83-100

Chetkowski, R.J., Meldrum, D.R., Steingold, K.A. *et al.* 1986. Biological effects of transdermal estradiol. *N Engl J Med,* **314**, 1615-20

Geola, F.L., Frumar, A.M., Tataryn, I.V. *et al.* 1980. Biological effects of various doses of conjugated oestrogens in post-menopausal women. *J Clin Endocrinol Metab,* **51**, 620-5

Guirguis, R.R. 1987. Oestradiol implants: what dose? how often? *The Lancet,* **ii**, 856

Steingold, K.A., Laufer, L., Chetkowski, R.J. *et al.* 1985. Treatment of hot flushes with transdermal estradiol administration. *J Clin Endocrinol Metab,* **61**, 627-32

Powers, M.S., Schenket, L., Carley, P.E. *et al.* 1985. Pharmacodynamics of transdermal dosage forms of 17B-oestradiol: comparison with conventional oral oestrogens used for hormone replacement. *Am J Obstet Gynecol,* **152**, 1099-106

Studd, J.W.W., Collins, W., Chakravarti, S. *et al.* 1977. Oestradiol and testosterone implants in the treatment of psychosexual problems in the post-menopausal woman. *Br J Obstet Gynaecol,* **84**, 314-15

Whitehead, M.I., Townsend, P.T., Pryse-Davies, J. *et al.* 1982. Effects of various types and dosages of progestogens on the post-menopausal endometrium. *J Reprod Med,* **27**, 539-48

Gambrell, R.D. & Massey, F.M. 1980. Use of progestogen challenge test to reduce the risk of endometrial cancer. *Obstet Gynecol*, **55**, 732-8

The prevention and treatment of endometrial pathology in post-menopausal women receiving exogenous oestrogens. 1980. In *The Menopause and Post-menopause*, eds. N. Pasetto, R. Paoletti, J.L. Ambrus, pp. 127-39. Lancaster, MTP Press

Staland, B. 1981. Continuous treatment with natural oestrogens and progestogens: a method to avoid hyperstimulation. *Maturitas*, **3**, 145-56

Magos, A.L., Brincat, M., Studd, J.W.W., Wardle, P., Schlesinger, P., O'Dowd, T. 1985. Amenorrhoea and endometrial atrophy with continuous oral estrogen and progestogen therapy in post-menopausal women. *Obstet Gynecol*, **65**, 496-9

Whitehead, M.I. 1986. Prevention of endometrial abnormalities. In *A Modern Approach to the Peri-menopausal Years*, ed. R.B. Greenblatt, pp. 189-206. Berlin, de Gruyter

Boston Collaborative Drug Surveillance Program. 1974. Surgically confirmed cases of gall-bladder disease, venous, thromboembolism and breast tumours in relation to post-menopausal estrogen therapy. *N Engl J Med*, **290**, 15-18

Gambrell, R.D. 1986. Prevention of endometrial cancer with progestogens. *Maturitas*, **8**, 159-68

Stanczyk, F.Z. 1989. Pharmacology of progestogens. *Int Proc J*, **1**, 11-20

Bush, T.L., Barrett-Connor, E., Cowan, L.D. *et al.* 1987. Cardiovascular mortality and non-contraceptive use of oestrogen in women: results from the Lipid Research Clinics program follow-up study. *Circulation*, **75**, 1102-9

Chez, R.A. 1989. Clinical aspects of three new progestogens: desogestrel, gestodene and norgestimate. *Am J Obstet Gynecol*, **160**, 1296-1300

Hammarback, S., Bäckstrom, C.T., Holst, J., Schoultz, B., Lyrenas, S. 1985. Cyclical mood changes as in the premenstrual tension syndrome during sequential estrogen-progestogen post-menopausal replacement therapy. *Acta Obstet Gynecol Scand*, **64**, 393-7

Vessey, M.P., Villard-Mackintosh, L., McPherson, K., Yeates, D. 1989. Mortality among oral contraceptive users: 20 years follow-up of women in a cohort study. *Br Med J*, **299**, 1487-91

Stampfer, M.J., Willett, W.C., Colditz, G.A., Speizer, F.E., Hennekens, C.H. 1988. A prospective study of past use of oral contraceptive agents and risk of cardiovascular diseases. *N Engl J Med*, **319**, 1313-17

Royal Australian Coll Ob & Gyn Bulletin. 1991. *Consensus statement on HRT and the menopause*, 19-20

Kloosterboer, H.J. 1990. Long-term effects of Org OD14 on lipid metabolism in post-menopausal women. *Maturitas*, **12**, 37-42

Tax, L. 1987. Clinical profile of Org OD14. *Maturitas* (suppl 1), 3-13

Crona, N. 1988. Treatment of climacteric complaints with Org OD14. *Maturitas*, **9**, 303-8

Bewley, S. & Bewley, T.H. 1992. Drug dependence with oestrogen replacement therapy. *The Lancet*, **339**, 290-1

Hulka, B.S. 1980. Effect of exogenous estrogen on post-menopausal women: the epidemiologic evidence. *Obstet Gynecol Surv*, **35**, 389-99

Adami, H.O., Persson, I., Hoover, R., Schairer, C., Bergkvist, L. 1989. The risk of cancer in women receiving hormone replacement therapy. *Int J Cancer*, **44**, 833-9

Hartge, P., Hoover, R., McGowan *et al.* 1988. Menopause and ovarian cancer. *Am J Epidemiol*, **1276**, 990-8

Cancer Research Campaign. 1991. *Factsheet 17*

Birkhauser, M.H., Hanggi, W. 1993. Benefits of different routes of administration. In *Abstract of the international symposium oon Women's Health in Menopause*, 26-29 September 1993. Milan

Riis, B.J., Jensen, J., Christiansen, C. 1987. Cyproterone acetate, an alternative gestagen in postmenopausal estrogen/gestagen therapy. *Clin Endocrinol*, **26**, 327-34

Tuppruainen, M., Saarikoski, S., Heikkinen, A.M., Honkanen, R., Kroger, H., Alhava, E., eds. 1993, Effect on bone density in osteoporotic women treated with a sequential combination of estradiol valerate 2 mg and cyproterone acetate 1 mg or calcitonin. *Proceedings of the 7th International Congress on the Menopause*, 20-24 June 1993, Stockholm

Christiansen, C., Riis, B.J. 1990 . Five years with continuous combined oestrogen/progestogen therapy. Effects on calcium metabolism, lipoproteins, and bleeding pattern. Br J Obstet Gynaecol, vol 97, 1087-92

Nielsen, S.P., Barenholdt, O., Hermansen, F., Munk-Jensen, N. 1994. Magnitude and pattern of skeletal response to long term continuous and cyclic sequential oestrogen/progestin treatment. *Br J Obstet Gynaecol*, vol 101, 319-24

Munk-Jensen, N. *et al*. 1994. Kliofem. *Am J Obstet Gynecol*, **171**, 132-8

Chapter 6 Cancer risk and the oestrogens used in HRT

[1] Harris, J.R., Lipmann, M.E., Veronesi, U., Willett, W. 1992. Breast cancer. (Review) *N Engl J Med*, **327**, 319-28

[2] Colditz, G.A. 1993. Epidemiology of breast cancer: findings from the Nurses' Health Study. *Cancer*, **71**, 1480-9

[3] Mansel, R.E. 1994. Breast Pain. ABC of Breast Diseases, *Br Med J*, **309**, 866-8

[4] Page, D.L., Steel, C.M., Dixon, J.M. 1995., Carcinoma in situ and Patients at High Risk of Breast Cancer. ABC of Breast Diseases, *Br Med J*, **310**, 39-41

[5] McPherson, K., Steel, C.M., Dixon, J.M. 1994. Breast Cancer – Epidemiology, Risk Factors, and Genetics. ABC of Breast Diseases, *Br Med J*, **309**, 1003-6

[6] Weber, J.A., May, P.E. 1989. Abundant class of human DNA/polymorphisms which can be typed using the polymerase chain reaction. *Am J Hum Genet*, **44**, 388-96

[7] Campagnoli, C., Biglia, N., Lanza, M.G., Lesca, L., Peris, C., Sismondi, P. 1993. Hepatocellular effects of progestogens used in hormone replacement treatment and breast cancer risk. In *Frontiers in Gynecologic and Obstetric Investigation*, ed. A.R. Genazzani, F. Petraglia, A.D. Genazzani. Carnforth: Parthenon Publ., 345-53.

[8] Campagnoli, C., Biglia, N., Lanza, M.G., Lesca, L., Peris, C., Sismondi, P. 1994. Androgenic progestogens oppose the decrease of insulin-like growth factor I serum level induced by conjugated oestrogens in postmenopausal women. *Maturitas*, **19** (1), 25-31

[9] Miller, V.T., Muesing, R.A., La Rosa, J.C., Stoy, D.B., Philips, E.A., Stillman, R.J. 1991. Effects of conjugated equine estrogen with and without three different progestogens on lipoproteins, high-density lipoprotein subfractions, and apolipoprotein A-I. *Obstet Gynecol*, **77**, 235-40

[10] Grady, D., Ernster, V. 1991. Does postmenopausal hormone therapy cause breast cancer? *Am J Epidemiol*, **134**, 1396-400

[11] Armstrong, B. 1988. Oestrogen therapy after the menopause: boon or bane? *Med J Aust*, **148**, 213-14

[12] Dupont, W.D., Page, D.L. 1991. Menopausal estrogen replacement therapy and breast cancer. *Arch Intern Med*, **151**, 67-72

[13] Steinberg, K.K., Thacker, S.B., Smith, J. *et al*. 1991. A meta-analysis of the effect of estrogen replacement therapy on the risk of breast cancer. *JAMA*, **265**, 1985-90

[14] Colditz, G.A., Egan, K.M., Stampfer, M.J. 1993. Hormone replacement therapy and risk of breast cancer. *Am J Obstet Gynecol*, **168**, 1473-80

[15] Sillero-Arenas, M., Delgado-Rodriques, M., Rodrigues-Cantera, R., Bueno-Cavanillas, A., Galves-Vargas, R. Menopausal hormone replacement therapy and breast cancer: a meta-analysis. *Obstet Gynecol*, **79**, 286-94

[16] Bergkvist, L., Adami, H.O., Persson, I., Hoover, R., Schairer, C. 1989. The risk of breast cancer after estrogen and estrogen-progestin replacement. *N Engl J Med*, **321**, 293-7

[17] Persson, I., Yuen., J., Bergkvist, L., Adami, H.O., Hoover, R., Schairer, C. 1992. Combined estrogen-progestogen replacement and breast cancer. *The Lancet*, **340**, 1044

[18] McPherson, K., Steel, C.M., Dixon, J.M. 1994. Breast Cancer – Epidemiology, risk factors, and genetics. ABC of Breast Diseases, *Br Med J*, **309**, 1003-6

[19] Early Breast Cancer Trialists' Collaborative Group. 1992. Systemic treatment of early breast cancer by hormonal, cytotoxic or immune therapy: 133 randomised trials involving 31,000 recurrences and 24,000 deaths among 75,000 women. *The Lancet*, **339**, 1-15, 71-85

[20] Seoud, M.A.-F., Johnson, J., Weed, Jr, J.C. 1993. Gynecologic tumours in tamoxifen-treated women with breast cancer. *Obstet & Gynecol*, **82**, no. 2, 165-9

[21] Jordan, V.C. 1993. How safe is tamoxifen? Only large randomised controlled trials can decide. *Br Med J*, **307**, 1371-2

[22] Masotti, L., Casali, E., Galeotti, T. 1988. Lipid peroxidation in tumour cells. *Free Radical Biol Med*, **4**, 377-86

[23] Halliwell, B. 1993. Free radicals and vascular disase: how much do we know? *Br Med J*, **307**, 885

[24] Sporn, M. Retinoids. *Oncology Rev*, **4**, 15-16

[25] Gambrell, R.D. 1986. Prevention of endometrial cancer with progestogens. *Maturitas*, **8**, 159-68

[26] Persson, I., Adami, H.O., Bergkvist, L. *et al*. 1989. Risk of endometrial cancer after treatment with oestrogens alone or in conjunction with progestogens: results of a prospective study. *Br Med J*, **298**, 147-51

[27] Ziel, H.K. 1982. Estrogen's role in endometrial cancer. *Obstet Gynecol*, **60**, 509-15

[28] Hulka, B.S. 1980. Effect of exogenous estrogen on post-menopausal women: the epidemiologic evidence. *Obstet Gynecol Surv*, **35**, 389-99

[29] Andersson, K., Mattsson, L.A., Rybo, G., Stadberg, E. 1992. Intrauterine release of levonorgestrel. A new way of adding progestogen in hormone replacement therapy. *Obstet Gynecol*, **79**, 963-7

[30] Adami, H.O., Persson, I., Hoover, R., Schairer, C., Bergkvist, L. 1989. The risk of cancer in women receiving hormone replacement therapy. *Br J Obstet Gynaecol*, **94**, 620-35

[31] Hartge, P., Hoover, R., McGowan *et al*. 1988. Menopause and ovarian cancer. *Am J Epidemiol*, **127**, 990-8

[32] Austoker, J. 1994. Screening for ovarian, prostatic, and testicular cancers. Cancer Prevention in Primary Care. *Br Med J*, **309**, 315-17

[33] Hunt, K., Vessey, M., McPherson, K., Coleman, M. 1987. Long-term surveillance of mortality and cancer incidence in women receiving hormone replacement therapy. *Br J Obstet Gynaecol,* **94,** 620-35

[34] Adami, H.O., Persson, I., Hoover, R., Schairer, C., Bergkvist, L. 1989. The risk of cancer in women receiving hormone replacement therapy. *Int J Cancer,* **44,** 833-9

[35] Machin, S.J., Mackie, I.J. 1993. Routine measurement of fibronogen concentration. Not clinically feasible. *Br Med J,* **307,** 882-3

[36] Gambrell, R.D. 1986. Prevention of endometrial cancer with progestogens. *Maturitas,* **8,** 159-68

[37] Persson, I., Adami, H.O., Bergkvist, L. *et al.* 1989. Risk of endometrial cancer after treatment with oestrogens alone or in conjunction with progestogens: results of a prospective study. *Br Med J,* **198,** 147-51

[38] Ziel, H.K. 1982. Estrogen's role in endometrial cancer. *Obstet Gynecol,* **60,** 509-15

[39] Hulka, B.S. 1980. Effect of exogenous estrogen on post-menopausal women: the epidemiologic evidence. *Obstet Gynecol Surv,* **35,** 389-99 ·

[40] Adami, H.O., Persson, I., Hoover, R., Schairer, C., Bergkvist, L. 1989. The risk of cancer in women receiving hormone replacement therapy. *Br J Obstet Gynaecol,* **94,** 620-35

[41] Hartge, P., Hoover, R., McGowan *et al.* 1988. Menopause and ovarian cancer. *Am J Epidemiol,* **127,** 990-8

[42] Hunt, K., Vessey, M., McPherson, K., Coleman, M. 1987. Long-term surveillance of mortality and cancer incidence in women receiving hormone replacement therapy. *Br J Obstet Gynaecol,* **94,** 620-35

[43] Adami, H.O., Persson, I., Hoover, R., Schairer, C., Bergkvist, L. 1989. The risk of cancer in women receiving hormone replacement therapy. *Int J Cancer,* **44,** 833-9

Chapter 7 Non-hormonal management of the menopause

Rebar, R.W. & Spitzer, I.B. 1987. The physiology and measurement of hot flushes. *Am J Obstet Gynecol,* **156,** 1284-5

Brincat, M., Versi, E., Moniz, C.F. *et al.* 1987. Skin collagen changes in post-menopausal women receiving different regimens of estrogen therapy. *Obstet Gynecol,* **70,** 123-7

Padwick, M.L., Whitehead, M.I., Coffer, A., King, R. 1988. Demonstration of oestrogen receptor related protein in female tissues. In *The Menopause,* eds. J.W.W. Studd & M.I. Whitehead, pp. 227-33. Oxford, Blackwell

Heaney, R.P. 1987. The role of nutrition in prevention and management of osteoporosis. *Clin Obstet Gynecol,* **50,** 833-46

Bell, N.H., Gosden, R.N., Henry, D.P., Shary, L., Epstein, S. 1988. The effects of muscle-building exercise on vitamin D and mineral metabolism. *J Bone Miner Res,* **3,** 369-73

Dalsky, G.P., Stocke, K.S., Ehsani, A.A., Slatopolsky, E., Lee, W.C., Birge, S.J. 1988. Weight-bearing exercise training and lumbar bone mineral content in post-menopausal women. *Ann Intern Med,* **108,** 824-8

Clarke, D.H. 1988. Training for strength. In *Women and Exercise, Physiology and Sports Medicine,* eds. M. Shangold & G. Mirken, pp. 55-64. Philadelphia, F.A. Davis

Fahey, T.D. 1988. Endurance training. In *Women and Exercise, Physiology and Sports Medicine,* eds. M. Shangold & G. Mirken, pp. 65-78. Philadelphia, F.A. Davis

Notelovitz, M., Fields, C., Caramelli, K., Dougherty, M., Schwartz, A.L. 1986. Cardio-respiratory fitness evaluation in climacteric women: comparison of two methods. *Am J Obstet Gynecol,* **154,** 1009-13

Heany, R.P., Gallagher, J.C., Johnstone, C.C. *et al.* 1983. Calcium nutrition and bone health in the elderly. *Am J Clin Nutr*, **36**, 986-1013

Sheikh, M.S., Santa Ana, C.A., Nicar, M.J., Schiller, L.B., Fordtran, J.S. 1987. Gastrointestinal absorption of calcium from milk and calcium salts. *N Engl J Med*, **317**, 532-6

Nicar, M.J. & Pak, C.Y.C. 1985. Calcium bioavailability from calcium carbonate and calcium citrate. *J Clin Endocrinol Metab*, **61**, 391-3

Delsay, J.L., Behall, K.M., Prather, E.S. 1979. Effect of fiber from foods and vegetables on metabolic responses of human subjects II. Calcium magnesium, iron and silicon balances. *Am J Clin Nutr*, **32**, 1876-80

Newcomer, A.D., Hodgson, S.F., McDill, D.B., Thomas, P.J. 1978. Lactase deficiency: prevalence in osteoporosis. *Ann Intern Med*, **89**, 218-20

Kleeman, C.R., Bohannan, J., Bernstein, D., Ling, S., Maxwell, M.H. 1964. Effect of variations in sodium uptake on calcium excretion in normal humans. *Proc Soc Exp Biol Med*, **115**, 29-32

Reichel, H., Koeffler, P., Norman, A.W. 1989. The role of vitamin D. Endocrine system in health and disease. *N Engl J Med*, **320**, 980-91

Howat, P.M., Varner, L.M., Hegsted, M., Brewer, M.M., Mills, C.Q. 1989. The effect of bulimia upon diet, body fat, bone density and blood components. *J Am Diet Assoc*, **89**, 929-34

Baron, J.A. 1984. Smoking and estrogen-related disease. *Am J Epidemiol*, **119**, 9-22

Frezza, M., di Padova, C., Pozzato, G. *et al.* 1990. High blood alcohol levels in women. *N Engl J Med*, **322**, 95-9

Wilson, R.C.D. 1983. Cardiovascular disease: prevention in practice. *BC Med J*, vol 25, **9**, 441-3

Wilson, R.C.D. 1989. Premenstrual syndrome. *Mod Med Can*, vol 44, **4**, 408-20

Chouinard, A. 1987. Unravelling the pathways and actions of hormones, essential fatty acids and opioids. *Can Med Assoc J* Oct, **137**, 593-6

Depression, inflammatory disease linked to oestrogen. *J Clin Invest* (US), October 1993

Chapter 8 Contraception and the menopause – present and future

Guillebaud, J. 1985. Contraception for the older woman. *J Obstet Gynaecol*, **5** (suppl 2), 570-7

Upton, G.V. 1988. Contraception in the woman over forty. In *The Menopause*, eds. J.W.W. Studd & M.I. Whitehead, pp. 289-304. Oxford, Blackwell

Trussell, J. & Westoff, C.F. 1980. Contraceptive practice and trends in coital frequency. *Fam Plan Perspect*, **12**, 246-9

Fioretti, P., Fruzzetti, F., Navalesi, R. *et al.* 1987. Clinical and metabolic study of a new pill containing 20 micrograms ethinylestradiol plus 0.15 mg desogestrel. *Contraception*, **35**, 229-43

Shargil, A.A. 1985. Hormone replacement therapy in peri-menopausal women with a triphasic contraceptive compound. A three-year prospective study. *Int J Fertil*, **30**, 15-28

Tayob, Y., Adams, J., Jacobs, H.S., Guillebaud, J. 1985. Ultrasound demonstration of increased frequency of functional ovarian cysts in women using progesterone-only oral contraception. *Br J Obstet Gynaecol*, **92**, 1003-9

Vessey, M.P., Lawless, M., McPherson, K., Yeats, D. 1983. Tubal sterilisation: findings in a large prospective study. *Br J Obstet Gynaecol*, **90**, 203-9

Magos, A.L., Brincat, M., Studd, J.W.W. *et al.* 1985. Amenorrhoea and endometrial atrophy with continuous oral estrogen and progestogen therapy in post-menopausal women. *Obstet Gynaecol,* **65,** 496-9

Drife, J.O. 1989. Complications of combined oral contraception. In *Contraception: Science and Practice,* eds. M. Filshie & J. Guillebaud, pp. 39-51. London, Butterworth

Vessey, M.P., Villard-Mackintosh, L., McPherson, K., Yeates, D. 1989. Mortality among oral contraceptive users: 20-year follow up of women in a cohort study. *Br Med J,* **200,** 1487-91

WHO Task Force on long-acting systemic agents for fertility regulation. 1988. A multicentred phase III comparative study of two hormonal contraceptive preparations given once a month by intramuscular injection: I. Contraceptive efficacy and side effects. *Contraception,* **37,** 1-20

WHO Task Force on long-acting systemic agents for fertility regulation. 1989. A multicentred phase III clinical study of two hormonal contraceptive preparations given once a month by intramuscular injection: II. The comparison of bleeding patterns. *Contraception,* **40,** 531-43

Folkman, J. & Long, D.M. 1964. The use of silicone rubber as a carrier for prolonged drug therapy. *J Surg Res,* **4,** 139-42

Segal, S.J. & Croxatto, H.B. 1967. *Single administration of hormones for long-term control of reproductive function.* Presentation at the XXIII meeting of the American Fertility Society. Washington DC

Mishell, D.R. & Lumkin, M.E. 1990. Contraceptive effect of varying dosages of progestogens in silastic vaginal rings. *Fertil Steril,* **21,** 99-103

Olsson, S.E. & Odlind, V. 1990. Contraception with a vaginal ring releasing 3-ketodesogestrel and ethinylestradiol. *Contraception,* **42,** 563-72

Odlind, V., Lithal, H., Kurunmaki, H. *et al.* 1984. ST 1435: development of an implant. In *Long-acting Contraceptive Delivery Systems,* eds., G.I. Zatuchni, A. Goldsmith, J. Shelton, J. Sciarra, pp. 441-9. Philadelphia, Penn, Harper & Row

Lähteenmaki, P. & Kurunmaki, H. 1984. Pharmacokinetic observations on ST 1435 administered subcutaneously and intravaginally. *Contraception,* **4,** 381-9

Darney, P.D., Monroe, S.E., Klaisle, C.M. *et al.* 1989. Clinical evaluation of the Capronor contraceptive: preliminary report. *Am J Obstet Gynecol,* **5,** 1291-5

Singh, M., Saxena, B.B., Landesman, R. *et al.* 1985. Contraceptive efficacy of bioabsorbable pellets of norethisterone (NET) as subcutaneous implants: phase II clinical study. *Adv Contracept,* **1,** 131-47

Luukkainen, T., Allonen, H., Haukkamaa, M., Lähteenmaki, P., Nilsson C.G., Toivonen, J. 1986. Five years' experience with levonorgestrel-releasing IUDs. *Contraception,* **33,** 139-48

Vessey, M.P. 1989. Oral contraception and cancer. In *Contraception, science and practice,* ed. M. Filshie, J. Guillebaud. London: Butterworth, 52-68

Guo, J., Wang, S-L, Wu, S-C. *et al.* 1990. Comparison of the clinical performance, contraceptive efficacy and acceptability of levonorgestrel-releasing IUD and Norplant-2 implants in China. *Contraception,* **41,** 485-94

Scholten, P.C., Christiaens, G.C.M.L., Alsbach, G.P.J. *et al.* 1989. Clinical experience with a levonorgestrel intrauterine device. In *The levonorgestrel IUD: Clinical performance and impact on menstruation,* ed. P.C. Scholten. Thesis. Utrecht, Netherlands

Luukkainen, T., Allonen, H., Haukkamaa, M. *et al.* 1987. Effective contraception with the levonorgestrel-releasing intrauterine device: 12-month report of a European multicenter study. *Contraception,* **36,** 169-79

Anderson, K., Mattson, L.A., Rybo, G., Stadberg, E. 1992. Intrauterine release of levonorgestrel: a new way of adding progestogen in hormone replacement therapy. *Obstet Gynecol,* **79,** 963-7

Liskin, L., Wharton, C., Blackburn, R. 1990. Condoms – now more than ever. *Population Repoorts.* Series H8, **18,** 1-36

Bounds, W., Guillebaud, J., Newman, G.B. 1992. Female condom (Femidon). A clinical study of its use-effectiveness and patient acceptability. *Br J Family Planning,* **18,** 36-41

Ford, N.J. 1992. Female condom improves with use. *Entre Nous,* **20,** 14

Drew, W.L., Blair, M., Miner, R.C. *et al.* 1990. Evaluation of the virus permeability of a new condom for women. *Sexually Transmitted Diseases,* **17,** 110-12

Chapter 9 Increased health risks at the menopause

Baines, C.J. 1987. Breast cancer screening: current evidence on mammography and implications for practice. *Can Fam Phys,* April, 33

Berkowitz, G.S. *et al.* 1985. Oestrogen replacement therapy and fibrocystic disease in post-menopausal women. *Am J Epidem,* **2,** 121

Lubin, F. *et al.* 1985. Overweight and changes in weight throughout adult life in breast cancer etiology. *Am J Epidem,* **4,** 122

Thompson, B., Hart, S.A., Durno, D. 1973. Menopausal age and symptomatology in a general practice. *J. Biosoc Sci,* **5,** 71-2

Bungay, G.T., Vessey, M.P., McPherson, K. 1980. Study of symptoms in middle life with special reference to the menopause. *Br Med J,* **281,** 181-3

Curtis, L.R., Curtis, G.B., Beard, M.K. 1986. *My Body – My Decision: what you should know about the most common female surgeries.* Tucson, Ariz., The Body Press

McPherson, K. *et al.* 1981. Regional variations in the use of common surgical procedures: within and between England and Wales, Canada and the USA. *Soc Sci Med,* **15A,** 273-88

Older, J. 1984. *Endometriosis: a woman's guide to a common but often undetected disease that can cause infertility and other major medical problems.* NY, Scribner

Reidel, H-H. *et al.* 1986. Ovarian failure after hysterectomy. *J Reprod Med,* July, **31,** 597-600

BMJ article. 1991. *The mysterious urethral syndrome.* 6 July, vol 303, 1

Ob Gyn Part 1. 1990. *CA125 levels in menopausal women.* Sept, vol 76, **3,** 428-31

BMJ article. 1991. *Sex hormones, autoimmune diseases and immune responses.* 6 July, vol 303, 2-3

Wright, V.C. 1989. Human papillomavirus infections. *Can Fam Phys,* June, vol 35, 1359-63

Mackel, J.V. & Krikke, E.H. 1989. Carcinoma of the cervix: an infectious disease?. *Can Fam Phys,* June, vol 35, 1353-7

The Guardian. 14 Sept 1990. Vaccine hope for cervical cancer virus

Managing the urogenital oestrogen deficiency syndrome. Sept 1991. Proceedings of the Novo Nordesk Symposium, Singapore

Beutner, K.R. 1990. Topical podofilox for treatment of condylomata acuminata in women. *Ob Gyn,* **76,** 656-9

Beutner, K.R. 1991. Clinical overview of podofilox for the treatment of anal/genital warts. *Proceedings of Dermatology,* Vancouver, Can

Cauwenbergh, G. 1988. Pharmacokinetic profile of orally administered itraconazole in the human skin. *JA Acad Derm*, **18** (2), 263-9

Cauwenbergh, G. 1991. New expectations in antifungal therapy. *Proceedings of Dermatology*, Vancouver, Can

Versi, E., Cardozo, L.D., Brincat, M., Cooper, D., Montgomery, J.C., Studd, J.W.W. 1988. Correlation of urethral physiology and skin collagen in postmenopausal women. *Br J Obstet Gynaecol*, **95**, 147-52

Versi, E., Cardozo, L.D., Studd, J.W.W., Brincat, M., O'Dowd, T.M., Cooper, D. 1986. Internal urinary sphincter in maintenance of female continence. *Br Med J*, **292**, 166-7

Fantl, J.A., Cardozo, L.D., McClish, D.K. 1994. Estrogen therapy in the management of urinary incontinence in postmenopausal women. A meta-analysis. *Obstetrics & Gynaecology*, **83**(1), 12-18

Hilton, P., Tweddel, A.L., Mayne, C. 1990. Oral and intravaginal estrogens alone and in combination with alpha adrenergic stimulation in genuine stress incontinence. *International Urogynaecology Journal*, **12**, 80-6

Cardozo, L.D., Rekers, H., Tapp, A. *et al.* 1993. Oestriol in the treatment of postmenopausal urgency: a multicentre study. *Maturitas*, **18**(1), 47-53

Associated Press and *The Guardian*, 9 February 1995

Genital Human Papillomavirus Infections. *ACOG Technical Bulletin*, no. 193, June 1994

Munoz, N., Bosch, F.X. de Sanjose, S. *et al.* 1992. The causal link between human papilloma virus and invasive cervical cancer: a population-based case-control study in Colombia and Spain. *Int J Cancer*, **52**, 743-9

Chapter 10 Common surgical procedures

Amerikia, H. & Evans, T.N. 1979. Ten-year review of hysterectomies: trends, indications and risks. *Amer J Obstet Gynecol*, **134**, 431-7

Cohen, S. & Soloway, R. 1985. *The Epidemiology of Gallstone Disease – Gallstones*. NY, Churchill-Livingstone

Harvard Medical School Health Letter. 1987. *Gallstones: are there alternatives to surgery?*. Aug, **12**, no 10

Payer, L. 1987. *How to Avoid a Hysterectomy: an indispensable guide to exploring your options before you consent to a hysterectomy*. NY, Pantheon

Weiss, N.S. & Harlow, B.L. 1986. Why does hysterectomy without bilateral oöphorectomy influence the subsequent incidence of ovarian cancer? *Amer J Epidem*, Nov., **5**, 124

Magos, A.L. (personal communication) April 1991. *Endometrial resection and HRT*

The Medical Post. 1990. Needle seen winning breast biopsy with knife, Feb., **20**, 46

Kirkpatrick, A.E. 1989. The radiological localisation of palpable lesions. *Current Imaging*, **1**, 108-13

Goldstein, S.R. 1994. Use of ultrasonohysterography for triage of perimenopausal patients with unexplained uterine bleeding. *Am J Obstet Gynecol*, **170**, 2, 565-70

Owens, S., Roberts, W., Fiorica, J., Hoffman, M., LaPolla, J., Cavanagh, D. 1989. Ovarian management at the time of radical hysterectomy for cancer of the cervix. *Gynecol Oncol*, **35**, 349-51

Ellsworth, L., Allen, H., Nisker, J. 1983. Ovarian function after radical hysterectomy for stage 1B carcinoma of the cervix. *Am J Obstet Gynecol*, **145**, 185-8

Jacobs, I., Oram, D. 1989. Prevention of ovarian cancer: A survey of the practice of prophylactic oöphorectomy by fellows and members of the Royal College of Obstetricians and Gynaecologists. *Br J Obstet Gynecol*, **96**, 510-15

Parker, M., Bosscher, J., Barnhill, D., Park, R. 1993. Ovarian management during radical hysterectomy in the premenopausal patient. *Obstet Gynecol*, **82**, 187-90

Chapter 11 Medical examinations and screening

Ferenczy, A. 1986. How to take and read Pap tests for the best patient management. *Contemporary OB/GYN,* May/June, 6

Thompson, D.W. 1989. *Adequate Pap smears: a guide for sampling techniques in screening for abnormalities of the uterine cervix.* Laboratory Proficiency Testing Program

Frisch, L.E., Parmar, H., Buckley, L.D. *et al.* 1990. Colposcopy of patients with cytologic inflammatory epithelial changes. *Acta Cytol*, **34**, 113

Ridgley, R., Hernandez, E., Cruz, C. *et al.* 1988. Abnormal Papanicolaou smears after earlier smears with atypical squamous cells. *J Reprod Med*, **33**, 285

Benedet, J., Boyes, D., Nichols, T. *et al.* 1976. Colposcopic evaluation of the patients with abnormal cervical cytology. *Br J Obstet Gynaecol*, **83**, 177

MacLelland, R. 1987. The essentials of screening mammography. *Cancer,* (suppl) **60**, 1678

Eddy, D.M., Hasselblad, V., McGirney, W. *et al.* 1988. The value of mammography screening in women under age 50 years. *J Am Med Assoc*, 259, 1512

Andersson, I., Aspegren, K., Janzon, L. *et al.* 1988. Mammographic screening and mortality from breast cancer: the Malmo mammographic screening trial. *Br Med J*, **297**, 943

Baines, C.J., Wall, C., Risch, H. *et al.* 1986. Changes in breast examination behavior in a cohort of 8214 women in the Canadian Breast Screening Study. *Cancer*, **57**, 1209

Tabar, L., Fagerberg, C.S.G., Day, N.E. 1988. The results of periodic one-view mammography screening in a randomised controlled trial in Sweden. Part 2: evaluation of results. In *Screening for Breast Cancer*, eds. N.E. Day & A.B. Miller, p. 39. Toronto, Huber

A statement by the British Society for Cervical Cytology and the British Society for Colposcopy and Cervical Pathology. 1991. *Cell content of cervical smears*

Boon, M.E. *et al.* 1986. Consequences of the introduction of combined spatula and cytobrush sampling for cervical cytology. *The International Academy of Cytology*, 1-5547

Reissman, S.E. 1988. Comparison of two Papanicolaou smear techniques in a family practice setting. *J Fam Practice*, vol 26, **5**, 525-9

Gilbertson, V.A. & McHugh, R. 1980. The earlier detection of colorectal cancers. A preliminary report of the occult blood study. *Cancer*, **45**, 2899-901

Hutchison, J. & Tucker, A.K. 1984. Breast screening results from a healthy working population. *Clinical Oncology*, **10**, 123 (Marks & Spencer)

Department of Health and Social Security. 1986. *Working group report to the health ministers of England, Wales, Scotland and Northern Ireland.* (Forrest Report) *Breast screening.* London, HMSO

UK trial of early detection of breast cancer group. First results on mortality reduction in the UK trial. 1988. *The Lancet*, **ii**, 411

Woodman, C.B.J., Threlfall, A.G., Boggis, C.R.M., Prior, P. 1995. Is the three-year breast-screening interval too long? Occurrence of interval cancers in NHS breast screening programme's north-western region. *Br Med J*, **310**, 224-6

Letters to *The Times*. Mr I. Fentiman, Deputy Director, Imperial Cancer Research Fund Clinical Oncology Unit, Guy's Hospital, London. 28 January 1995

NHS Breast Screening Programme. 1993. Review. Sheffield: NHS BSP, 1993

Semiglazov, V.F., Moiseyenko, V.M., Bavli, J.L., Migmanova, Nsh, Selznyov, N.K., Popova, R.T. *et al.* 1992. The role of breast self-examination in early breast cancer detection (results of the 5 years USSR/WHO randomised study in Leningrad). *Eur J Epidemiol,* **8,** 498-502

Beral, V. 1993. Breast cancer. Mammographic screening. *The Lancet,* **341,** 1509-10

Day, N.E. 1991. Screening for breast cancer. *Br Med Bull,* **47,** 400-15

Mant, D. 1992. Should all woman be advised to practise regular breast self-examination? *The Breast,* **1,** 108

Sutton, G.C., Balmer, S. 1994. Screening for breast cancer. Letters to Editor. *Br Med J,* **309,** 664

Field, S., Michell, M.J., Wallis, M.G.W., Wilson, A.R.M. What should be done about interval breast cancers? *Br Med J,* **310,** 203-4

Jen, J., Hoguen, K., Piantadosi, S. *et al.* 1994. Allelic loss of chromosome 18q and prognosis in colorectal cancer. *New Engl J Med,* **331,** 213-21

Chapter 12 Fifty years on – the future

Follicle xenografting. *Proceedings of 8th Reinier de Graaf Symposium: 'Ovarian Endocrinopathies',* Amsterdam, September 1993 Excerpta Medica

Gene therapy, *Financial Times,* 14 March 1995

INDEX